# Scottish Hospitals

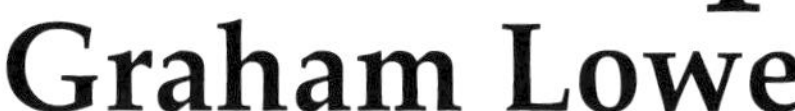

## Graham Lowe

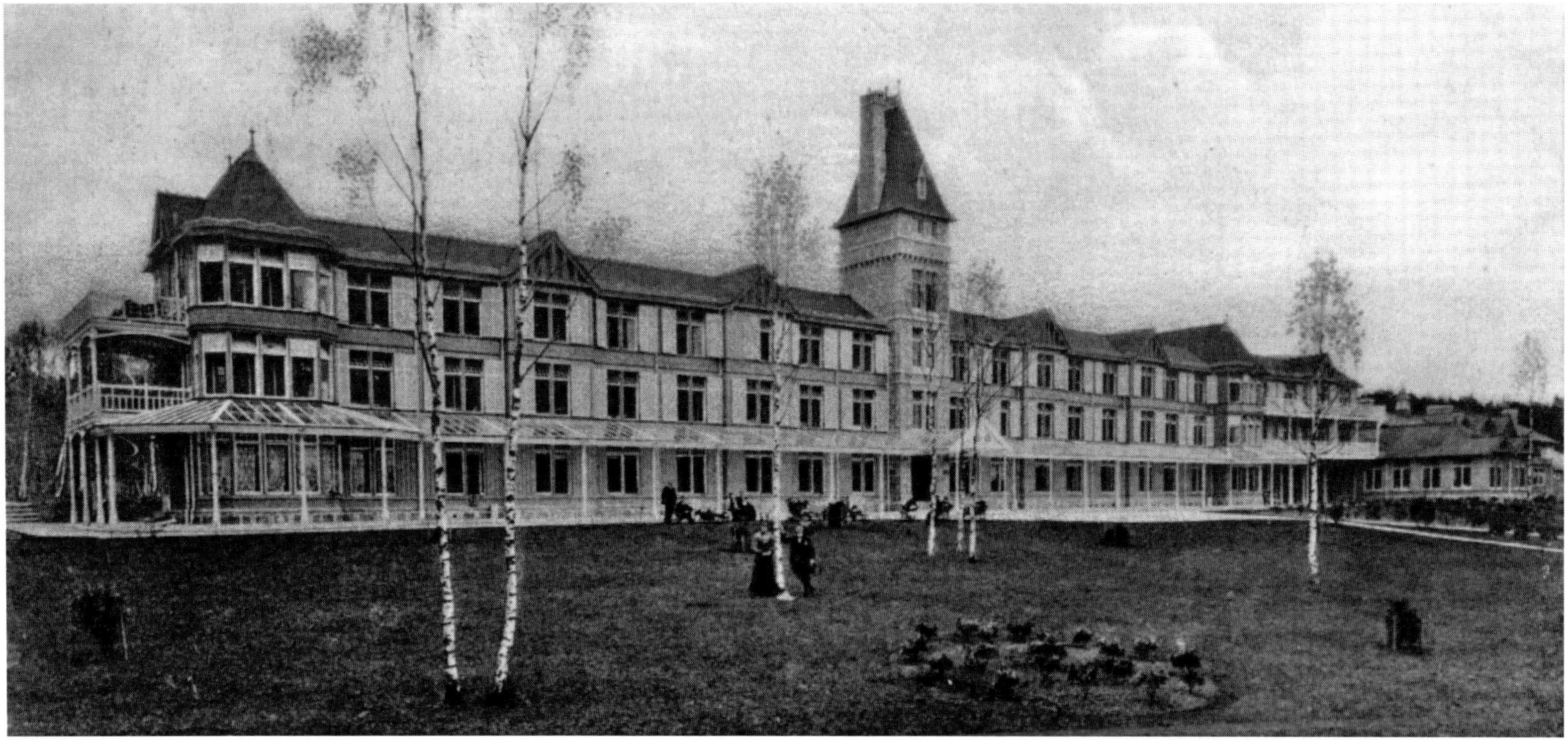

The Sanatorium in Banchory was built in 1900 as a private tuberculosis sanatorium, the first to be built in Scotland on the fresh air principle, and was named Nordrach-on-Dee after the Black Forest site in southern Germany where open-air treatment of TB was started by Dr Otto Walther in 1889. The windows could be kept open in all weathers to let in the scent of pine, which was thought to be beneficial. Beds rose from 36 to 75, but demand later subsided and closure came in 1928. It was converted into Glen O'Dee luxury hotel in 1934 and sold to the Red Cross at the end of the war, during which the hotel had been requisitioned by the army. It was returned to its original tuberculosis use in 1949, but with demand again dwindling it became an NHS convalescent hospital, with 78 beds in 1973. It later became a home for the elderly, closing in 1998, and a new community hospital was built on the same site. The original hospital, which was constructed mainly of timber, was destroyed by fire in 2016.

First published in the United Kingdom, 2018,
by Stenlake Publishing Ltd.
54-58 Mill Square, Catrine, KA5 6RD
www.stenlake.co.uk
ISBN 978-1-84033-804-1



Printed by
Berforts, 17 Burgess Road, Hastings, TN35 4NR

# Acknowledgements

I must pay tribute to my daughter Claire, who helped me in the early days of my postcard collection, although I did ask her to stop buying cards, just in case we were bidding against each other on Ebay!

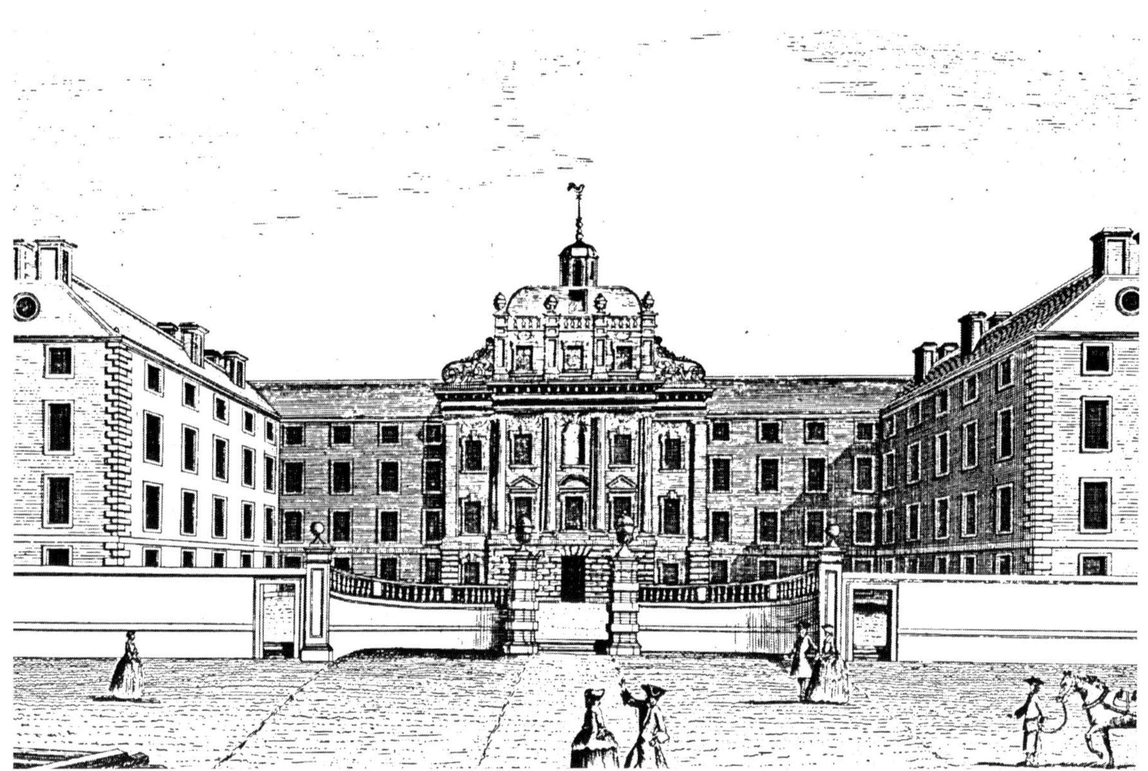

William Adams 1741, Edinburgh Royal Infirmary

# Scottish Hospitals

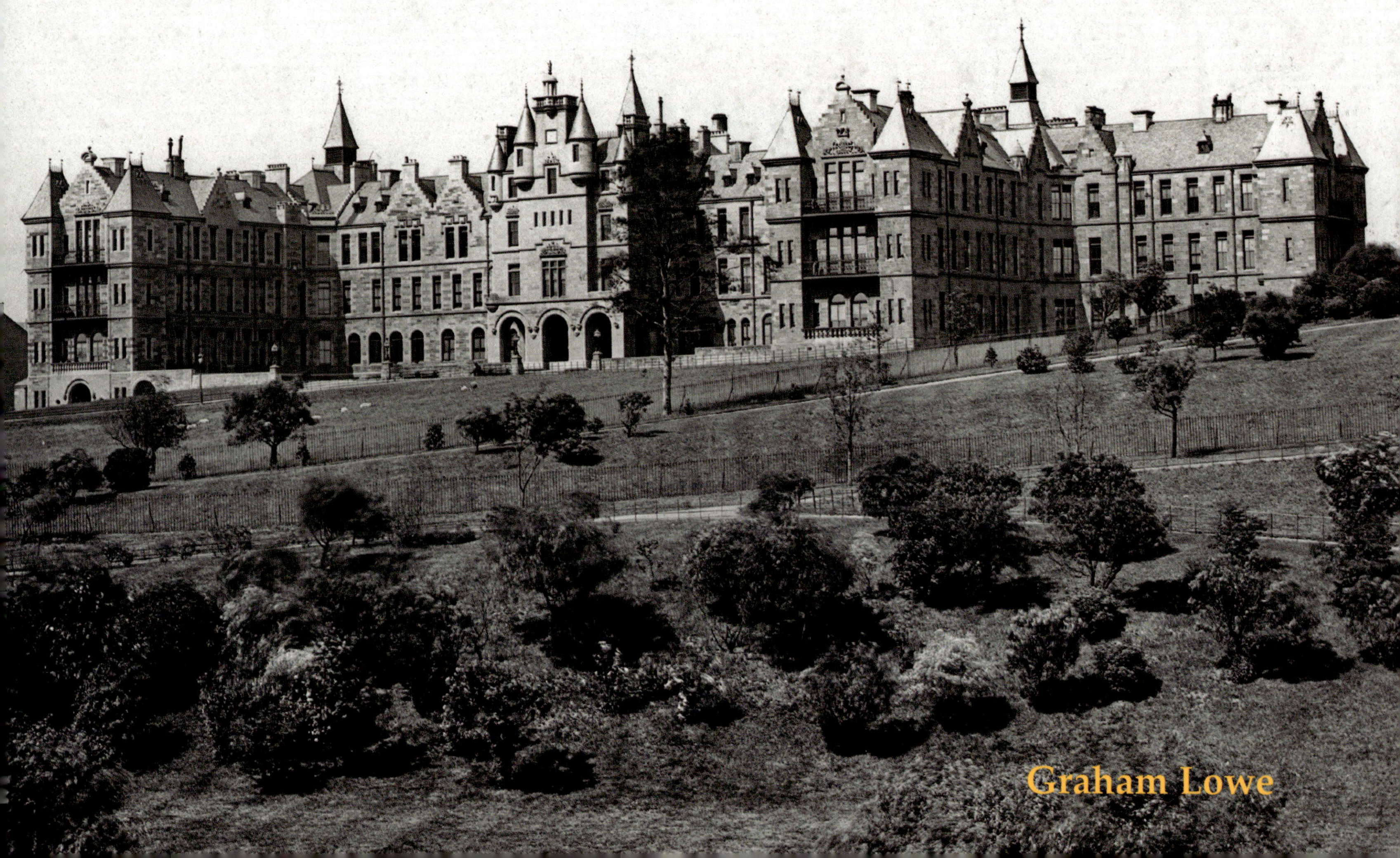

Graham Lowe

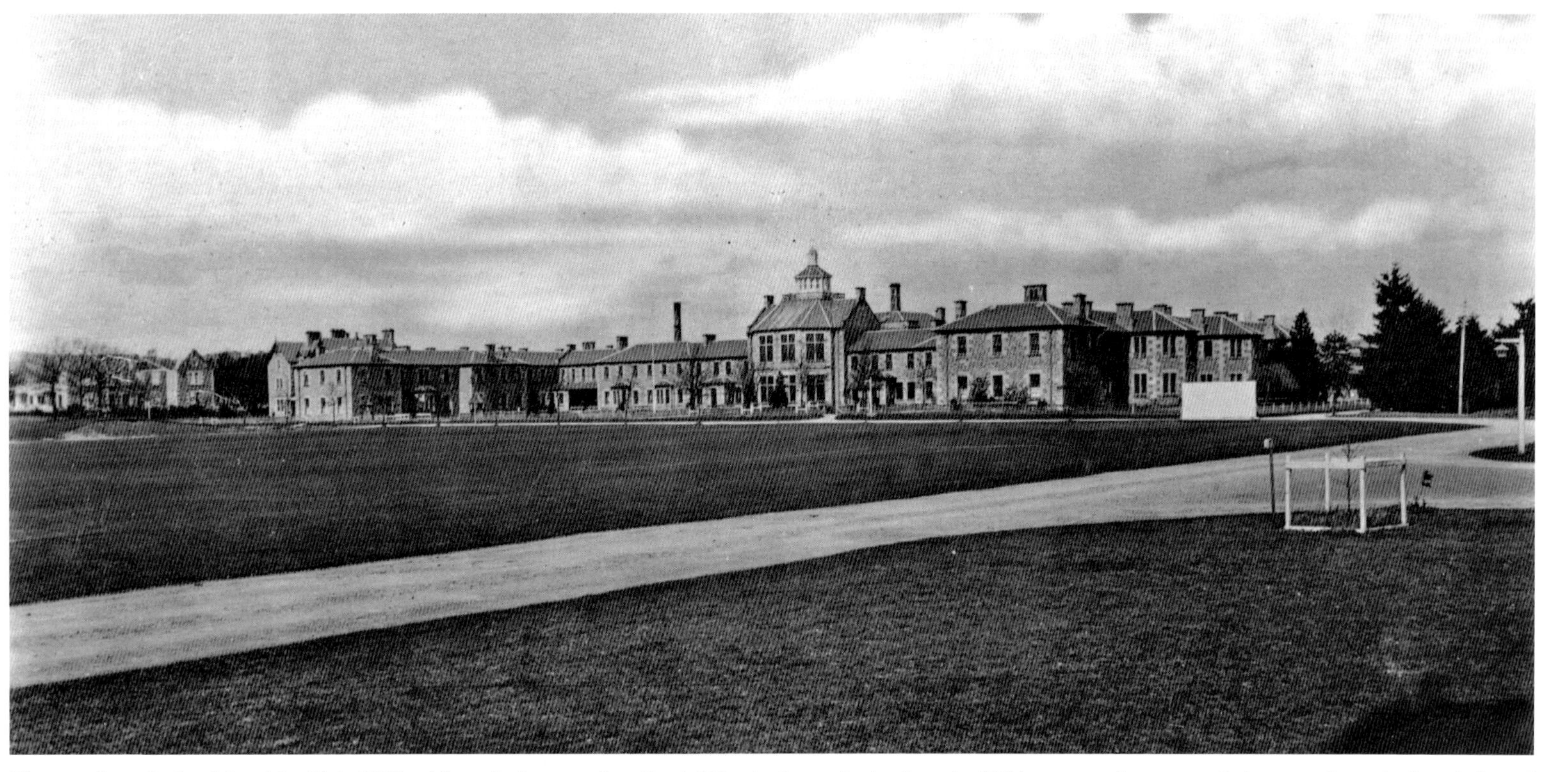

The war hospital at Murthly. This 222 bed hospital opened as Perth District Lunatic Asylum in 1864 to treat the county's 'pauper lunatics' and closed in 1984 as Murthly Psychiatric Hospital. During the First World War it was used as a war hospital providing beds for 350 other ranks, and was also used as a military psychiatric hospital from 1917 to 1919, the civilian patients being moved to other local psychiatric hospitals. It is likely that cases of shellshock were treated here.

*Front cover*: The Western Infirmary in Glasgow was planned and built as an integral part of the removal of Glasgow University from the High Street to Gilmorehill. This John Burnet-designed 'pavilion-style' infirmary opened as a voluntary hospital in 1874, its initial 150 beds rising to 630 by 1911. Sir William Macewen moved from the Royal to the Western when he became Regius Professor of Surgery (founded in 1815 by King George III) in 1892, and became the first to complete a successful surgical removal of the lung. The close physical relationship to the University emphasised its importance as a teaching hospital, and its research capacity increased with the opening of the Gardiner Institute of Medicine in 1938, taking its name from the family that gifted £25,000 towards its foundation; important research on atheroma, and adrenal and renal mechanisms in high blood pressure, heart failure and Addison's disease took place under the auspices of the Medical Research Council after the Second World War. With the growth of medical and surgical specialities after the war a two phase rebuilding programme was authorised in 1964, but after Phase I was completed in 1974 Phase II was postponed indefinitely after nearby Gartnavel General Hospital was completed, and the Infirmary closed in 2015. The building is set to be redeveloped by the University, to include a pioneering Centre for Health and Wellbeing.

# Introduction

In medieval times, hospitals existed in Scotland, but were generally church-driven and designed to provide care for the poor, aged and chronically disabled rather than for patients with acute illness. After the Reformation practically no new hospitals were founded in Scotland until the voluntary hospital movement gradually gained momentum in the 18th century. This philanthropic enterprise arose from an intricate combination of factors, different parts of the country having their own particular driving force of necessity, inter-civic rivalry or charitable intent. Fund-raising came in many forms from public subscriptions, wealthy benefactors, church collections and all manner of social events, with particular support coming from the working class who had their own self-help ethos stimulated by dangerous work conditions of the time. Subscribers were granted privileges dependent on the amount of their donation, with all being able to recommend candidates for admission. In a voluntary hospital the visiting surgeons and physicians gave their services for free or for a nominal sum, earning their livelihoods in general or private practice outside the hospital. The voluntary movement only came to an end when the National Health Service arrived in 1948.

In the early days of the voluntary hospitals, most patients were poor, as anyone with enough money would normally have procured medical attendance within their own home. However, with the advent of anaesthesia, antisepsis and easily cleaned 'pavilion-style' wards with their cross-ventilation and separation / segregation of patients, hospitals were seen as safer places to have operations and be investigated, and gradually became no longer the preserve of the poor. By the end of the 19th century, an increasing complexity of ancillary buildings such as boiler rooms, x-ray suites, laundries, mortuaries, out-patient buildings and nurses homes were needed, and medical and nursing students had to be taught in the bigger hospitals. Medical knowledge was expanding, treatments were improving and hospital buildings were becoming better suited to their function.

The first section of this book gives an overview and examples of general voluntary hospitals which as the name implies catered mainly for general medical and surgical patients; these range in size from the large city teaching hospitals, through medium sized district general hospitals to smaller cottage hospitals. These are followed by examples of infectious diseases (fever) hospitals, tuberculosis sanatoria, hospitals for 'incurable' patients, Poor Law Hospitals, hospitals for special purposes, convalescent hospitals and wartime hospitals. Psychiatric hospitals are not included in this book.

For general voluntary hospitals, top of the pile in terms of hierarchy come the teaching hospitals of the university cities. As teaching hospitals, they play a predominant role in the clinical education of medical and nursing students. Smaller but no less important are the district general hospitals, which like the teaching hospitals provide a wide range of services, and also often contribute to clinical teaching and training. The smallest are the cottage hospitals providing a more limited range of services; some of these are a bit larger in size although not fulfilling the criteria of district general hospitals, unless rebuilt on a larger scale. Cottage hospitals are more commonly known nowadays as community hospitals, where most patients are admitted and cared for by their own GP who can deliver acute medical care where the expertise of a specialist hospital is not required, rehabilitation, casualty and palliative care services. Some of the larger hospitals have acquired the term 'Royal' in their title indicating some form of Royal Patronage, with perhaps some legal rights in addition.

In the early and mid 19th century, fever cases were sometimes randomly mixed in the general wards with non-fever cases, whereas others segregated the two or were accommodated in separate hospitals; a questionnaire sent by Dundee Royal Infirmary to several hospitals around the UK in the 1840s had shown a disturbing lack of unanimity on this practice. This was not solved until all areas built infectious disease hospitals which local authorities were responsible for providing following the 1889 Public Health Act; some areas used voluntary hospitals for these cases initially, but it was made compulsory after a further 1897 Act and infectious disease hospitals then proliferated around the country, sometimes in association with tuberculosis sanatoria when they were known as combination hospitals. Sanatoria on their own started to appear after Robert Koch discovered the tubercle bacillus as the cause of tuberculosis in 1882. As the original need for both these hospital types lessened in the 1950s with centralisation and better treatments becoming available, many of them changed function to provide care for the elderly, chronic sick, or convalescence.

Hospitals for incurables began to be established in the mid 19th century, welcomed by some and condemned by others; they met a need for those above the poverty line (those dependent on parish poor relief were ineligible for admission), and would admit the likes of cancer, rheumatism, paralysis, deformity and spinal disease which were less welcome in general hospitals because of the length of time they occupied the ward, the 'bed-blockers' of their day. The priority of these hospitals was to keep the patients comfortable and free from pain, although day rooms, libraries, smoking rooms, easy access to open air, lifts and wide corridors for wheelchairs were all to be welcomed.

Hospitals built by Parish Councils were there for the very poor of the district and were often built beside the poorhouses. They came under local authority control following a Government Act in 1929 which abolished Scottish Parochial Boards. Municipal hospitals run by local authorities were a product of the welfare system created by historic Poor Law legislation; in many people's eyes this also carried the stigma of the workhouse, although some tried hard to upgrade their services.

In 1870, there were just seven convalescent hospitals in Scotland providing short-term care for two to three weeks after surgery, trauma or illness. By the 1930s the number had increased to over 60, but sponsors now included hospitals, independent promotors, Co-operative and friendly societies and religious and temperance organisations and there was some blurring between the need for recuperation after illness and having a rest or a holiday. Nowadays, there are plenty of care homes at a price, but the NHS focus is on multidisciplinary rehabilitation and respite and palliative care provided at community hospitals and day care centres by teams of nurses, occupational therapists, speech therapists and physiotherapists.

During the First World War, casualties were accommodated in civil hospitals of all sizes and military hospitals, and dotted around the country there were a large number of auxiliary hospitals prepared by the Red Cross and other voluntary effort, often occupying large country houses; these were generally preferred by the troops as the discipline was not as strict as in the military hospitals, conditions were less crowded and the surroundings were more homely. By the end of the war there were all told 24,291 equipped hospital beds for officers and other ranks in Scotland.

The enormous casualty lists of the First World War were still a vivid memory when plans for building large numbers of temporary hospitals were drawn up in the Second World War, as the expectation was that there would be heavy civilian casualties from bombing. As well as the existing hospitals and requisitioned houses and hotels, seven large Emergency Medical Service hospitals were rapidly built to a standard design several miles from large centres of population, although close to the railway network to facilitate transport and transfer of casualties; in the event, there was less need in Scotland than anticipated for hospital care of air raid casualties, but these large hospitals served in many other ways right through into NHS days, although only Stracathro Hospital in Angus remains in use today.

Readers will note bed numbers and functions at the hospital opening, in wartime (meaning here the Second World War unless otherwise specified), in 1973 and now, designed to show changing trends over time. I have included where possible details of what has become of the old hospitals and what have replaced them (sometimes just a pile of rubble). Figures have been taken from a 1940s Scottish Home and Health Department report on future provision of hospital care, a 1973 NHS Directory of Scottish Hospitals, the internet and telephone. Any inaccuracies are of course my own.

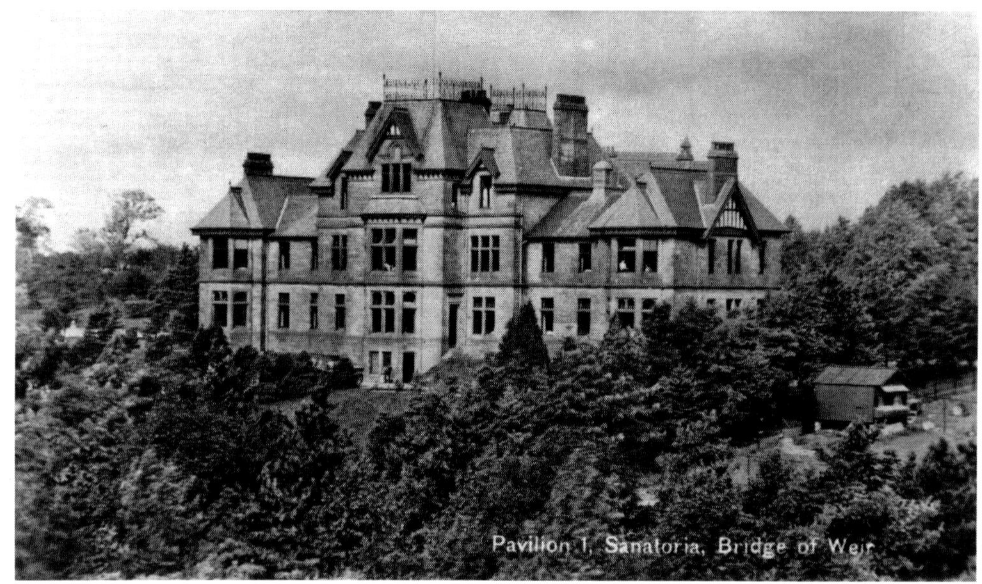


One of the three sanitoria pavilions in Bridge of Weir.

# Voluntary hospitals – Teaching hospitals

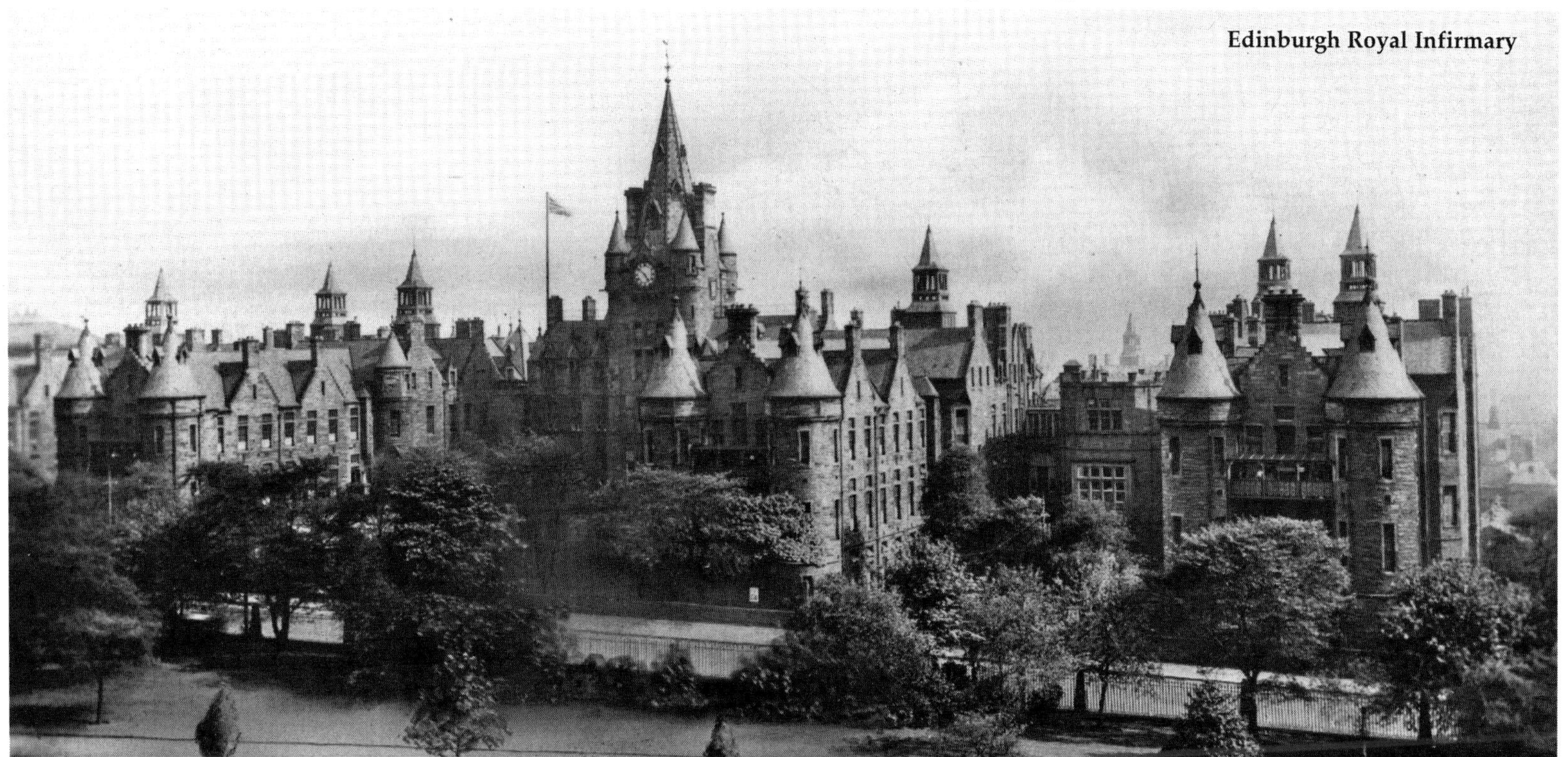

Edinburgh Royal Infirmary

Edinburgh Royal Infirmary began as a modest four bed hospital in 1729 which was followed by the first purpose-built hospital in Scotland designed by William Adam and built in 1741 as the Royal Infirmary of Edinburgh; its 228 beds were augmented later by two surgical units in 1832 and 1853. However, due to overcrowding the architect David Bryce was asked to design a new Royal Infirmary and his plans were heavily influenced by the 'pavilion model' being advanced by the nursing pioneer Florence Nightingale who was a miasmatist (a belief in 'bad air' or miasms as the cause of disease); this model was dependent on the rationale that with improved ventilation due to free circulation of light and air between the pavilions the mortality rate would significantly reduce, which it did. Designed in Scottish Baronial style, the new Infirmary (seen above) was opened at Lauriston Place in 1879, and Adam's Infirmary Street building was demolished five years later. Additions in the form of pavilions built in different styles to the original made their appearance from time to time, and there were 974 beds in 1973. By the 1990s it was widely recognised that the old-fashioned Infirmary was in urgent need of replacement, and the phased 900 bed move to Little France was finally completed in 2003, with a small part of Lauriston remaining to care for patients. Notable achievements in this Infirmary include Sir Michael Woodruff and James Ross performing the first successful living kidney transplant in the UK on identical twins in 1960, and Desmond Julian setting up Europe's first coronary care unit in 1964.

## Aberdeen Royal Infirmary

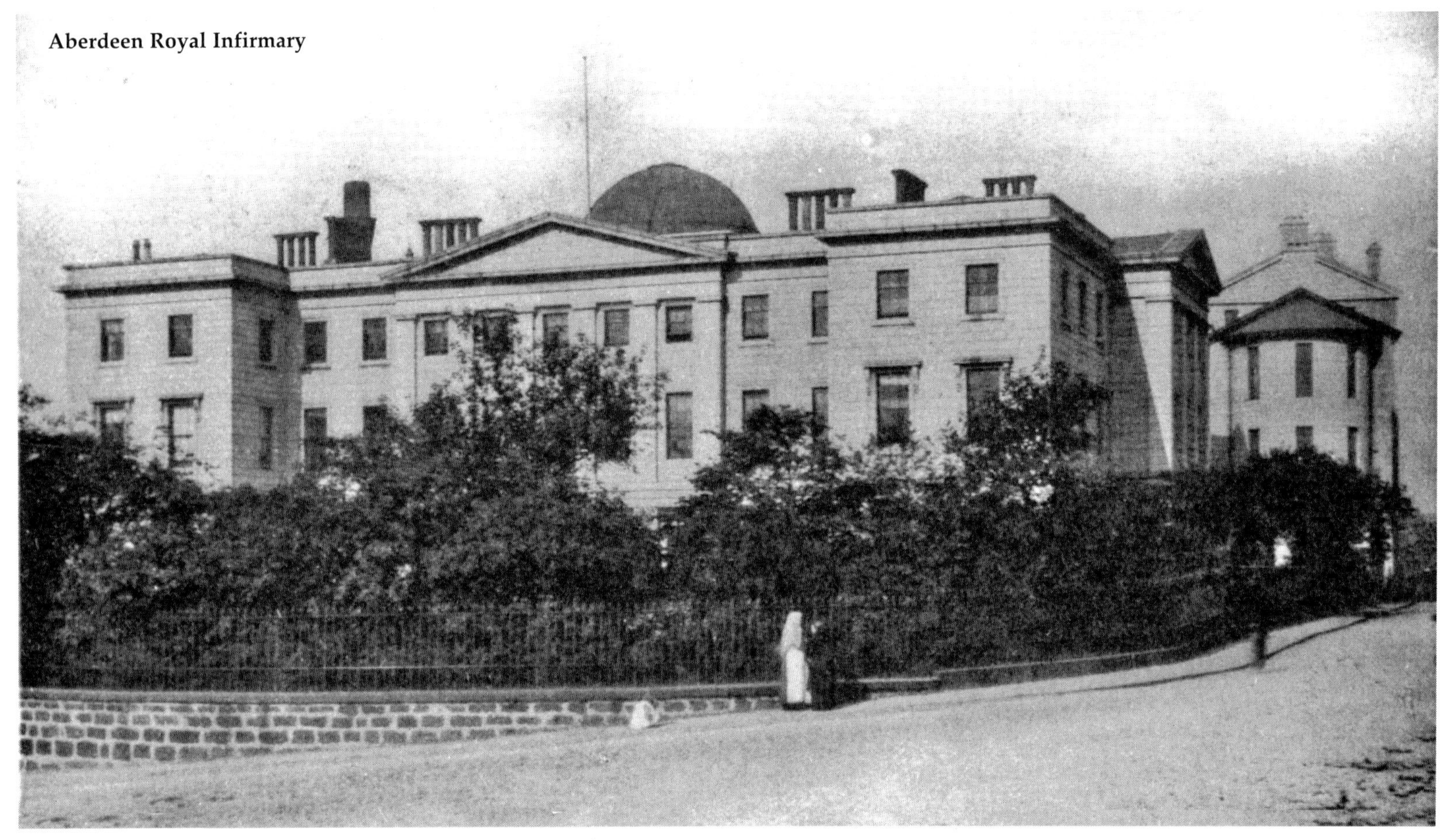

Aberdeen Royal Infirmary had its origin in 1742 at Woolmanhill with a small 20 bed hospital. It was enlarged in 1753, 1760 and 1820, with Royal Patronage coming in 1773. In 1840 it was rebuilt on the same site as an elegant neoclassical domed building designed by Archibald Simpson with 210 beds. The Infirmary was extended in 1897 and 1912, but then ran out of space and a large grey granite hospital complex was added on a new site in 1936; built at the elevated Foresterhill site on the outskirts of Aberdeen, this was a bold concept in design by James Brown Nicol linking general, maternity and children's hospitals on the same site as the medical school. There were 504 beds in wartime, 708 in 1973 and there are currently 922; additions have been such that the original complex of buildings is now hard to distinguish. Woolmanhill in the centre of Aberdeen remained in use as a hospital until 2017. The Infirmary is most famous for pioneering work on MRI scanning in the 1970s, and the world's first scanner went on display at its Foresterhill home in 2016. The photograph above shows Simpson's 1840 Woolmanhill building.

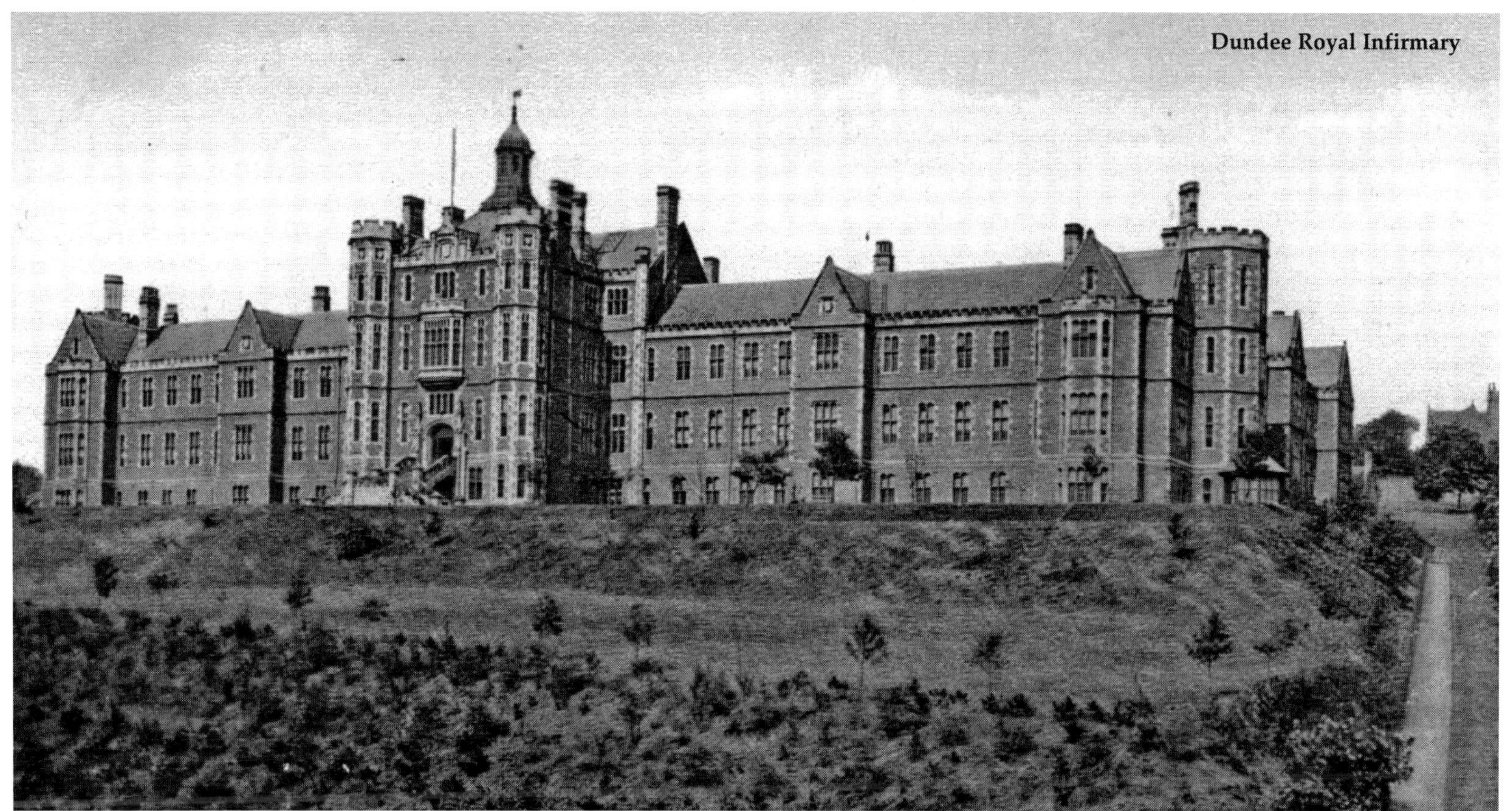

Dundee Royal Infirmary

When the first 1798 Dundee Royal Infirmary ran out of space, advice was sought from Professors Christison and Syme in Edinburgh on what to do next, and they came out in favour of a new build. The Tudor-style Royal Infirmary seen here designed by Coe and Goodwin of London opened in 1855. It was built in the declining years of the 'corridor plan' (where the wards opened off corridors) with high wards and awkwardly-placed side and accessory rooms, so quickly became out of date; the closely-following 'pavilion plan' with its cross-ventilated wards was associated with a sharp decline in hospital mortality rates, but DRI just missed out on this. Adjacent maternity and cancer wings were of more successful design, but gradually further disordered building filled up the site. After the Second World War when there were 449 beds, it was decided to build a new teaching hospital on the city outskirts, somehow losing Royal patronage in the process. A notable event came in 1967 with Lowe, Emslie-Smith and Watson's intracardiac research finding evidence of conduction in an important nerve bundle within the heart which led to a flurry of work in America, and in time to ablative treatment of heart conduction defects. Infirmary patients moved to the 862 bed Ninewells Hospital and Medical School in two stages, 1974 and 1998, and DRI subsequently redeveloped for housing.

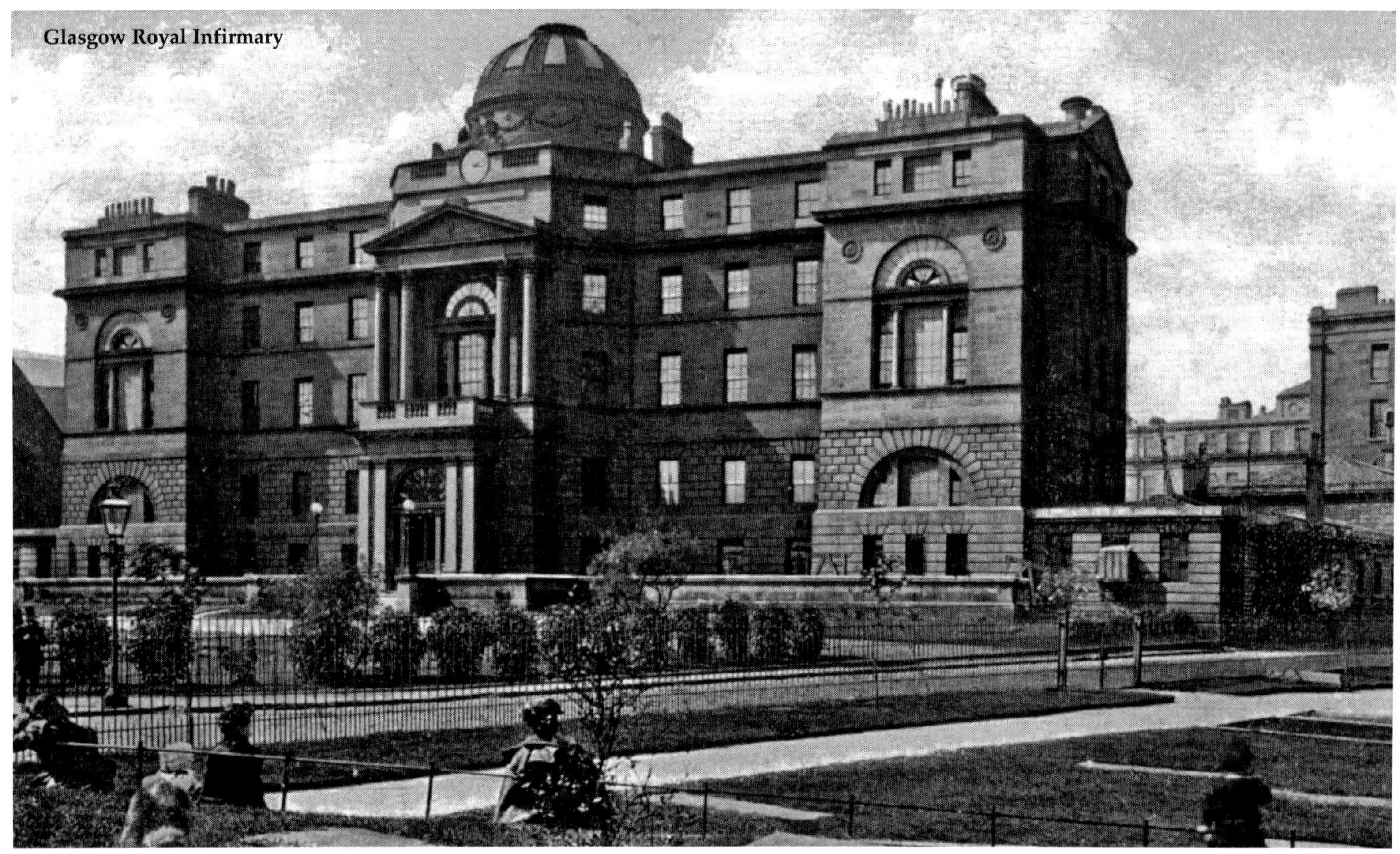


The Robert and James Adam-designed neoclassical Glasgow Royal Infirmary, adjacent to Glasgow Cathedral, opened in 1794 as a dignified expression of civic pride, accommodating 136 beds and a circular operating room on the fourth floor with a glazed dome ceiling. An extension in 1815, a separate fever house and Lister's surgical house brought the bed complement to over 600 by 1861. Notable achievements at the Infirmary include Joseph Lister evolving the principles of antiseptic surgery in 1867, William MacEwen introducing the practice of doctors wearing sterilisable white coats and being the first to surgically remove a brain tumour in 1879, and John McIntyre opening the first X-Ray department in the world in March 1896 just four months after Roentgen's discovery.

# Glasgow Royal Infirmary

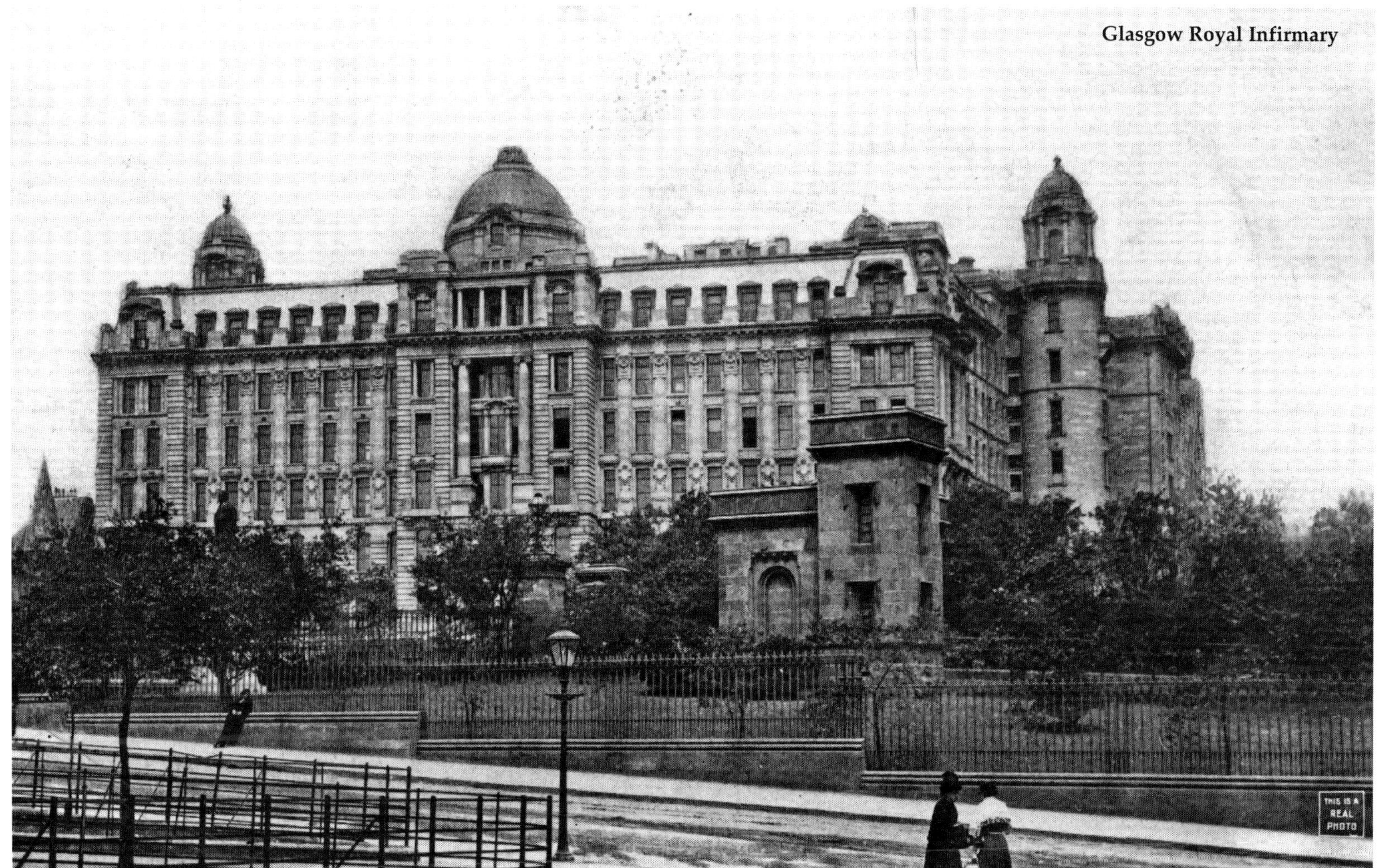


When it was decided to rebuild the Infirmary to commemorate Queen Victoria's Diamond Jubilee, James Miller was chosen as the architect but work proceeded slowly amidst disputes over the merits of the plans, in particular the height of the building which dwarfed the Cathedral, and the bulky building, seen above, was only eventually completed in 1914. The modern Queen Elizabeth building designed by Sir Basil Spence was completed in 1982, and this large teaching hospital now accommodates 1,077 beds.

# Voluntary hospitals – District general hospitals

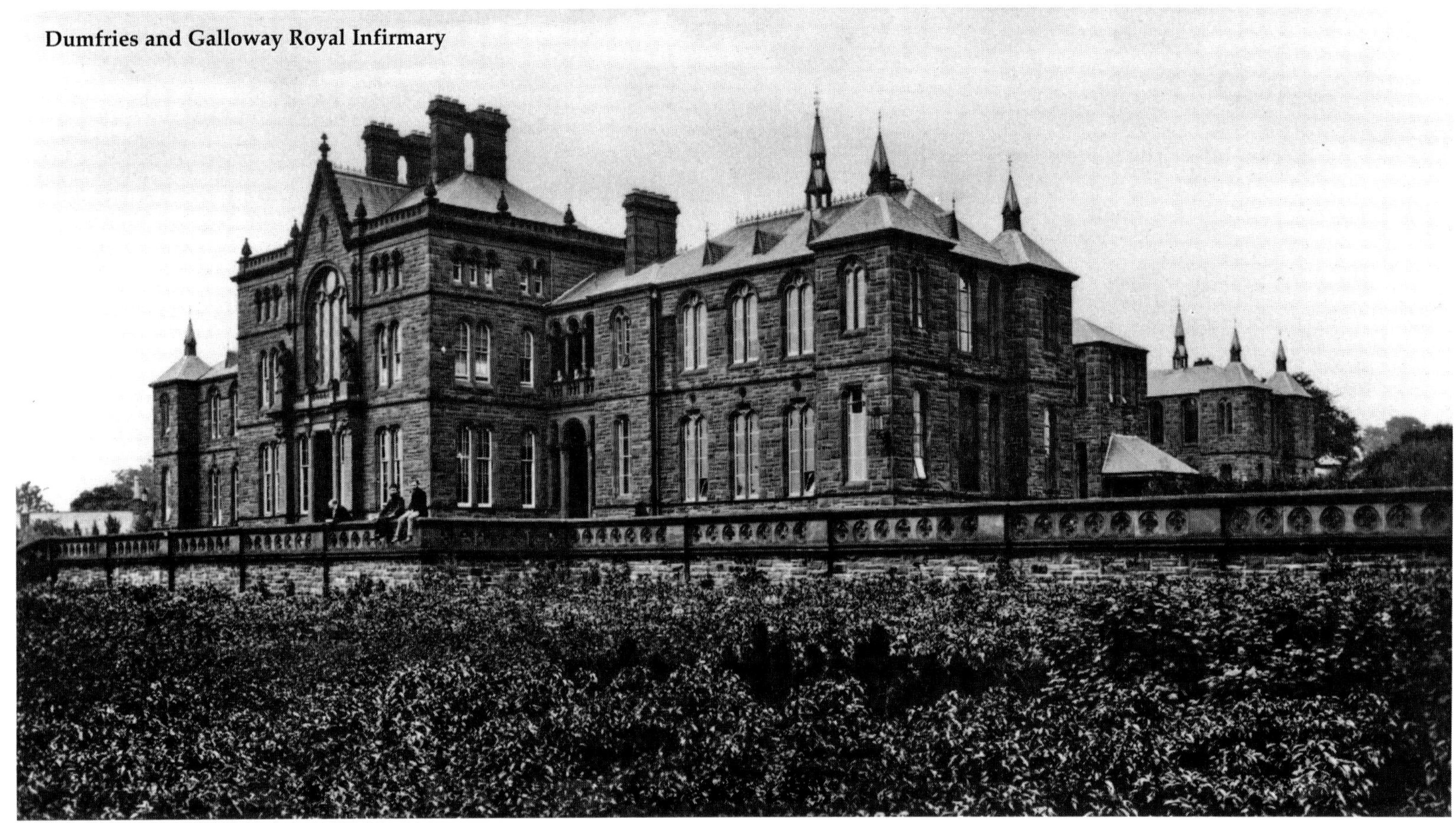

Dumfries and Galloway Royal Infirmary

The original modest Dumfries and Galloway Infirmary was built in 1778 and acquired Royal patronage in 1807; it is claimed that it was here that in 1846 Dr. William Scott became the first doctor in the UK to administer ether as a general anaesthetic. A new 170 bed Italianate-style hospital, designed by John Starforth on the 'pavilion plan', was built of red sandstone at Nithbank in 1873; flanking the main entrance were finely carved figures of Aesculapius the Greco-Roman god of medicine, and Hygeia goddess of health and daughter of Aesculapius. However, by the Second World War it was recognised that its general design no longer satisfied modern requirements for medical care, and so it was replaced by a new Infirmary in 1975 with a current bed complement of 337. This photograph is of Starforth's 1873 hospital, which now comprises an office for Dumfries and Galloway Health Board.

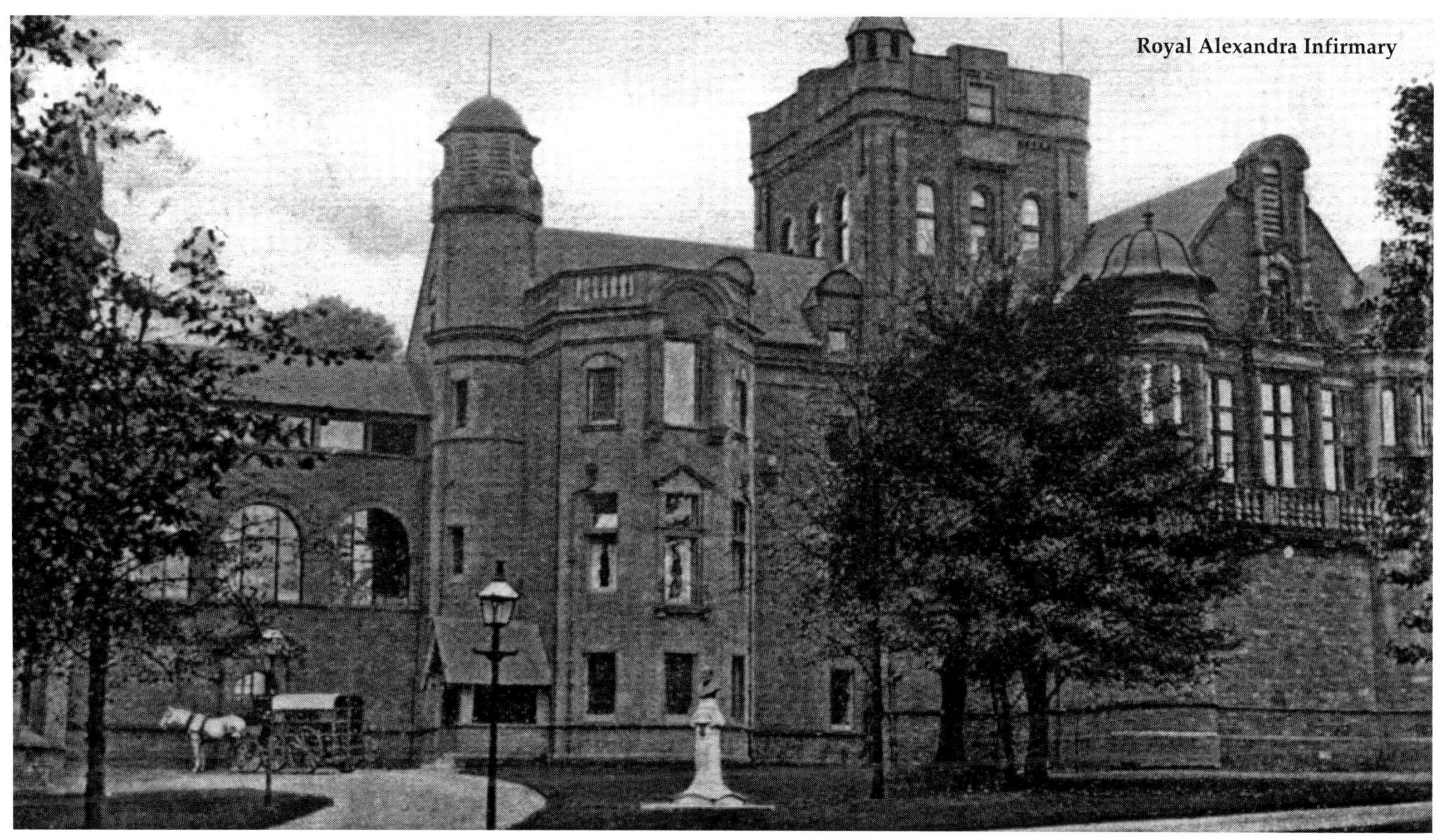

Royal Alexandra Infirmary

The first hospital in Paisley was a House of Recovery in 1805 for infectious diseases until 1850, when it became a general hospital with medical and surgical wards called Paisley Infirmary and Dispensary. It was rebuilt on a new greener site in 1900 and renamed as the Royal Alexandra Infirmary; richly endowed by the trustees of William B. Barbour and local mill owner Peter Coats, the very fine red sandstone infirmary shown here was designed by TG Abercrombie in Scottish Renaissance style. It incorporated circular wards to maximise light in a three-storey block to the north, with three ward pavilions to the south terminating in semi-circular open verandas to allow fresh air access and to harmonise the design, which also included an infectious diseases block. Various additions brought the bed complement up to 220 by wartime. The Infirmary closed in 1987 when a rebuilt 650 bed Royal Alexandra Hospital again opened on a new site. Part of the old Infirmary became a care home which closed in 2008 and it was otherwise flatted, but other parts are in a ruinous state.

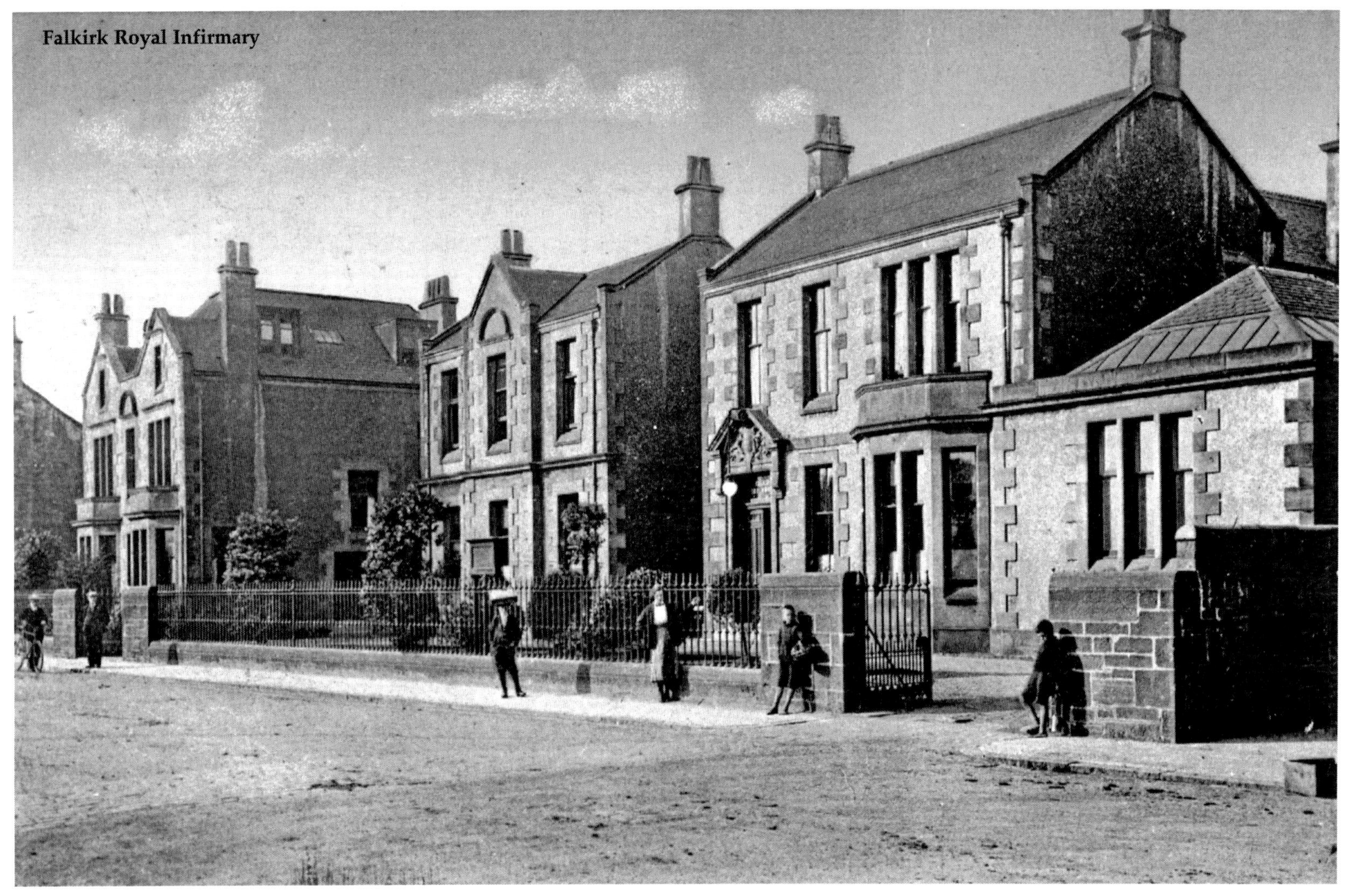


Falkirk Royal Infirmary started small and grew to be a 'Royal'. A cottage hospital opened in 1889, funded by public subscription, and this became Falkirk Infirmary in 1904. A new Infirmary became necessary due to growth in demand, and the local inhabitants seriously set about fund-raising, a 'grand bazaar' alone netting £10,000.

# Falkirk Royal Infirmary

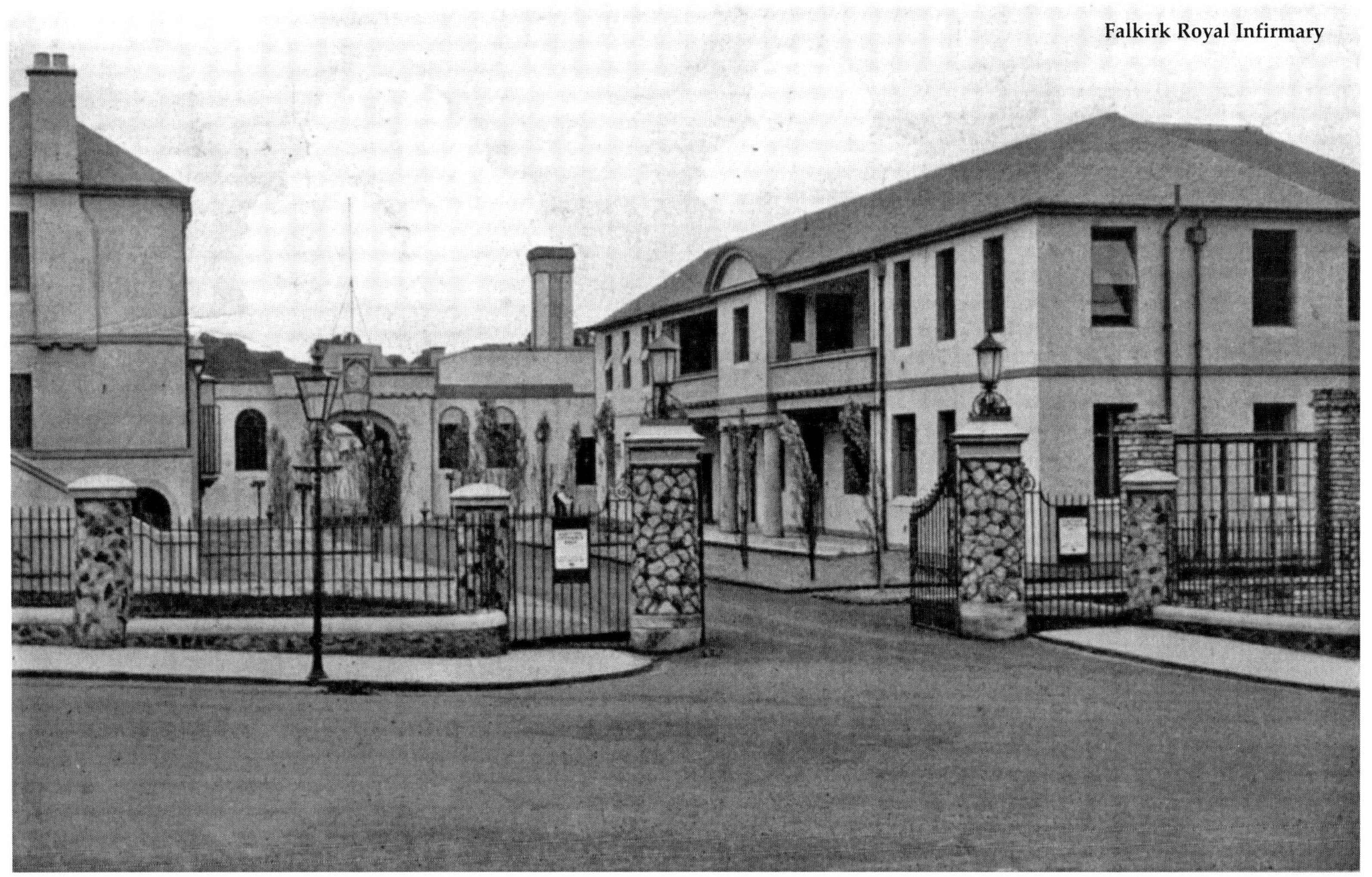

The opening ceremony of the now Falkirk Royal Infirmary in 1932 attracted 20,000 people, and despite costing £120,000, the 85 bed Infirmary opened free of debt; it is easy to imagine the immense feeling of pride that the Infirmary must have engendered amongst the local population. Within five years there were 200 beds and by 1973 there were 417. To local dismay however, the Infirmary was largely bulldozed in 2012 when patients moved to the controversial Private Finance Initiative 860 bed £300 million Forth Valley Royal Hospital at Larbert.

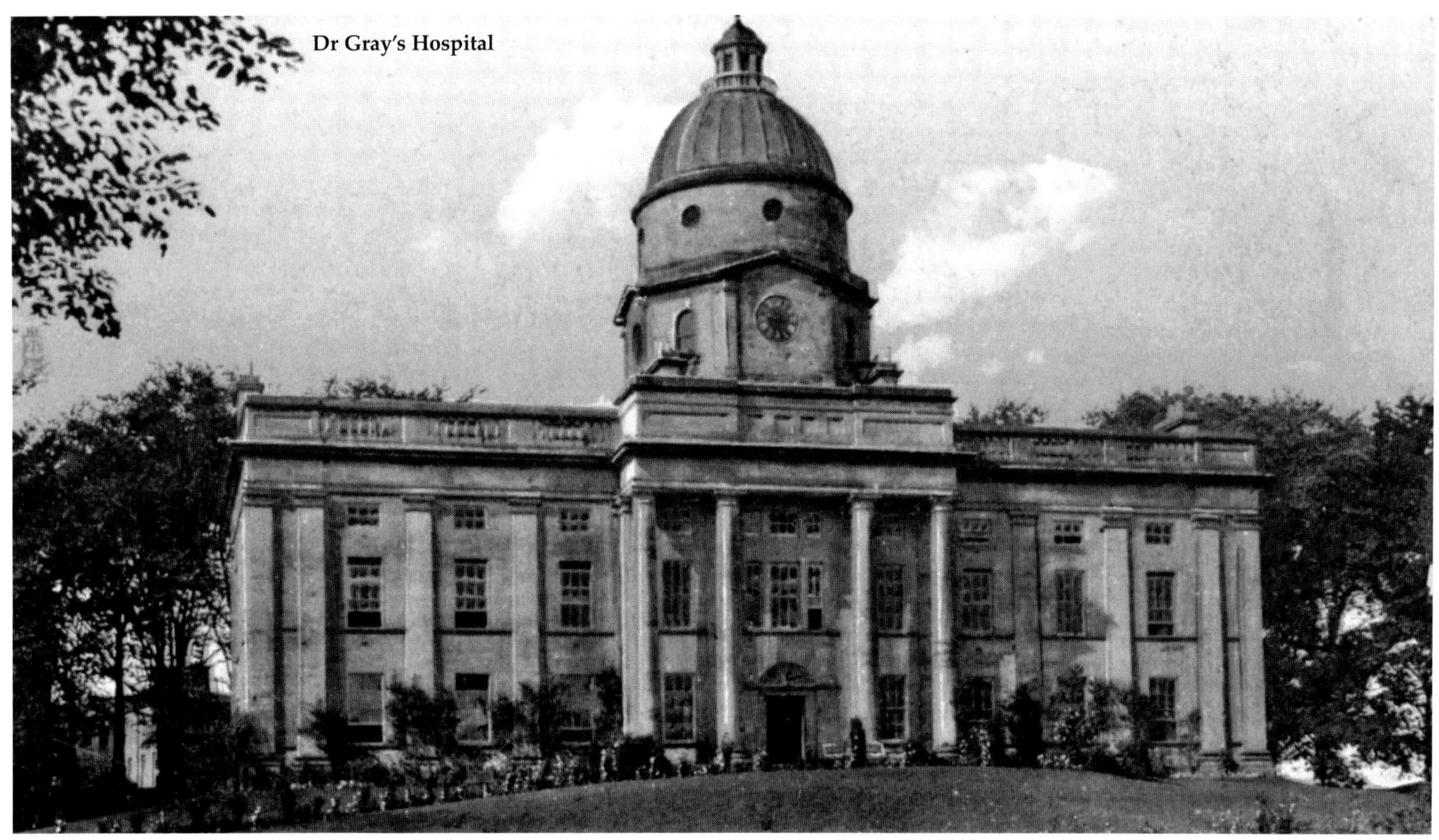
Dr Gray's Hospital

Dr. Gray's Hospital takes its name from Alexander Gray of Elgin, who spent 20 years in Bengal as a surgeon for the East India Company. He left £20,000 for the hospital, which opened in 1819 with 30 beds.The elegant classical building with giant Doric columns and topped with drum tower and dome was designed by James Gillespie Graham in the tradition of the grand civic statement, and the foundation stone ceremony was interrupted by news of Wellington's victory over Napoleon at Waterloo to double the celebrations of that day. By 1850 the upper floor was converted into fever wards which had a separate staircase entrance at the back of the building, but by the end of the century the local authority acknowledged their statutory responsibility by building a new infectious diseases hospital. Dr Gray's took in military patients in both World Wars; in WWI, it complemented the First Scottish General Hospital in Aberdeen as a treatment centre, nursing back to health over 900 casualties. Major redevelopment in the 1990s saw bed complement rising from post-WWII 60 to 185, Dr Gray's becoming the smallest district general hospital in Scotland, serving a population of over 70,000.

# Voluntary hospitals – Larger cottage hospitals

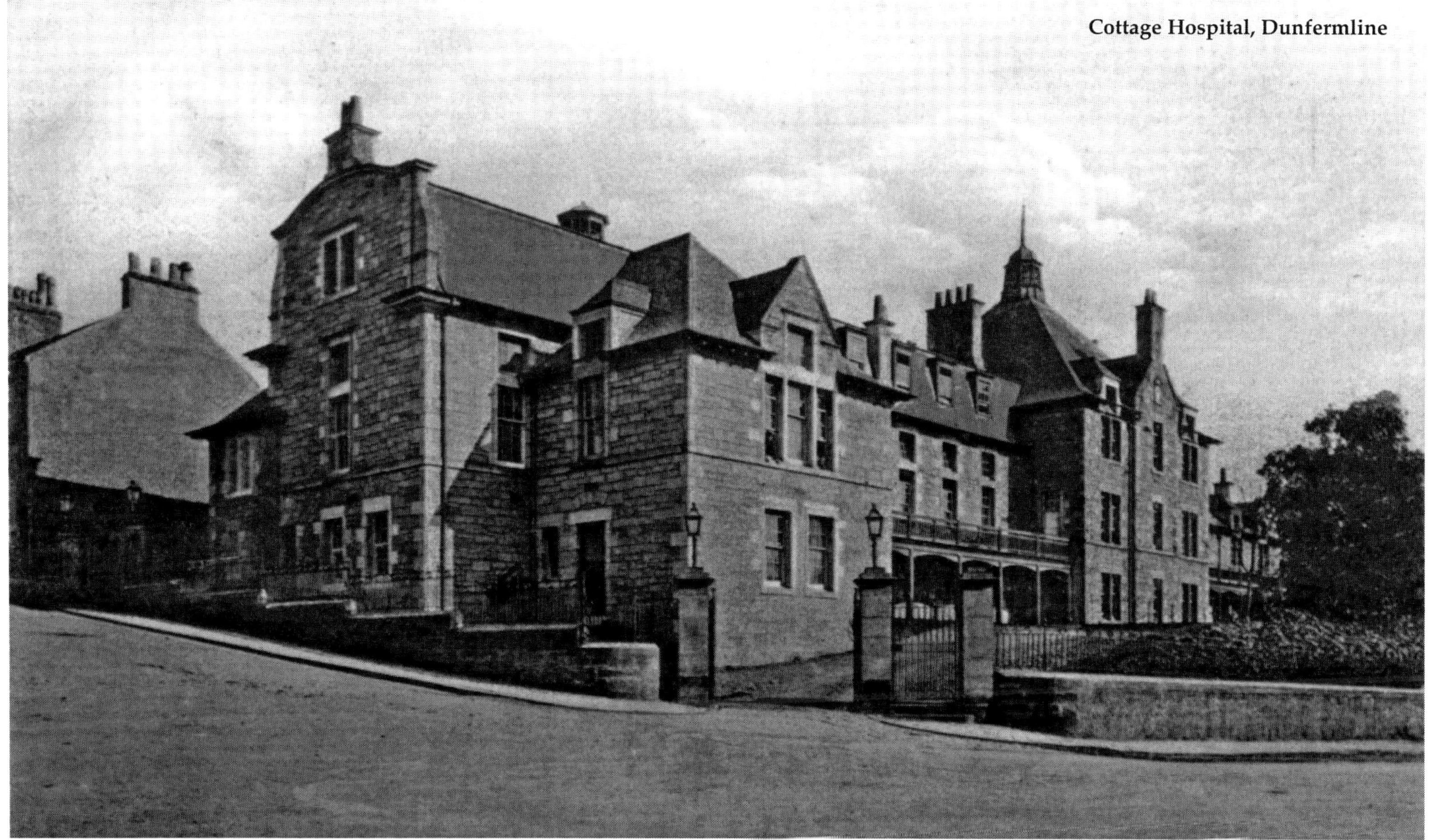

Cottage Hospital, Dunfermline

Dunfermline Cottage Hospital opened as a 16 bed cottage hospital in 1894, it was extended in 1898, 1904 and 1931 so that by wartime, and by then known as Dunfermline and West Fife Hospital, it had a complement of 100 beds. No charge was made at that time for hospital treatment but donations were asked for, and freely given; an exception was made for x-rays where a small charge was made, other than from miners and their dependants. A casualty block was a further addition in the 1950s, but the hospital became a crowded jumble of buildings on a restricted site and was mostly demolished after the 367 bed Queen Margaret Hospital was commissioned in 1985, with New City House being erected as council offices around the old hospital core in 2004.

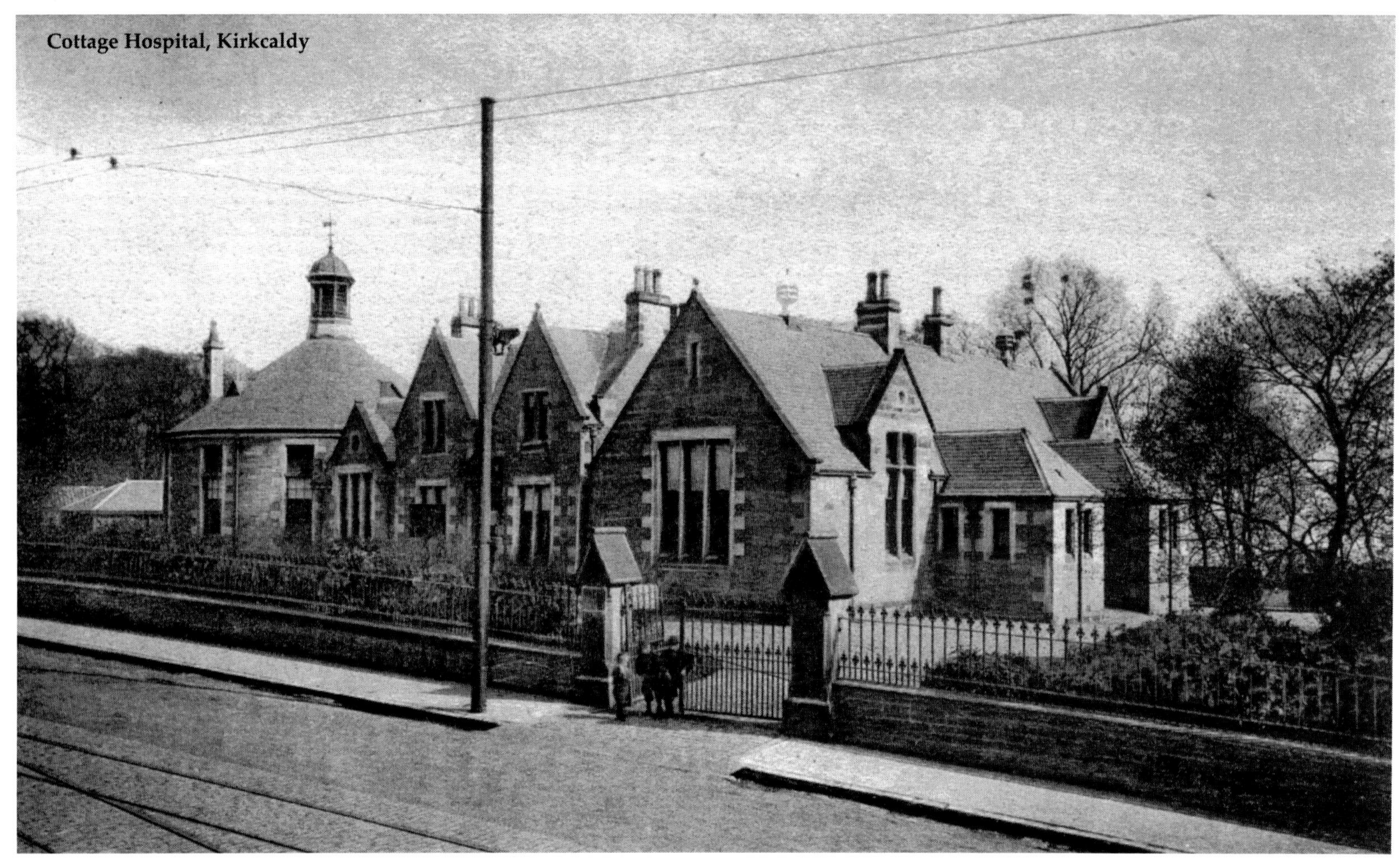
Cottage Hospital, Kirkcaldy

Sir Michael Nairn of the local floor cloth weavers had Kirkcaldy Cottage Hospital built on a site next to Ravenscraig Castle. It opened in 1890 with ten beds and underwent extension in 1895 and 1914 to become the only cottage hospital in Scotland to have a circular ward, designed by Gillespie and Scott of St. Andrews and copied from the original ward plans of Johns Hopkins Hospital in Baltimore. Additions were made from time to time so that by wartime, when it was known as Kirkcaldy General Hospital and by locals as the Auld General Hospital, the complement had become 74 beds. The hospital was replaced in 1967 by the Victoria Hospital with its 14 storey ward tower and 458 beds. Shortly before demolition in 1984, a lady dressed in grey was seen by children gliding through the corridor weeping; it is unknown who she is or whether she haunts the former hospital or castle.

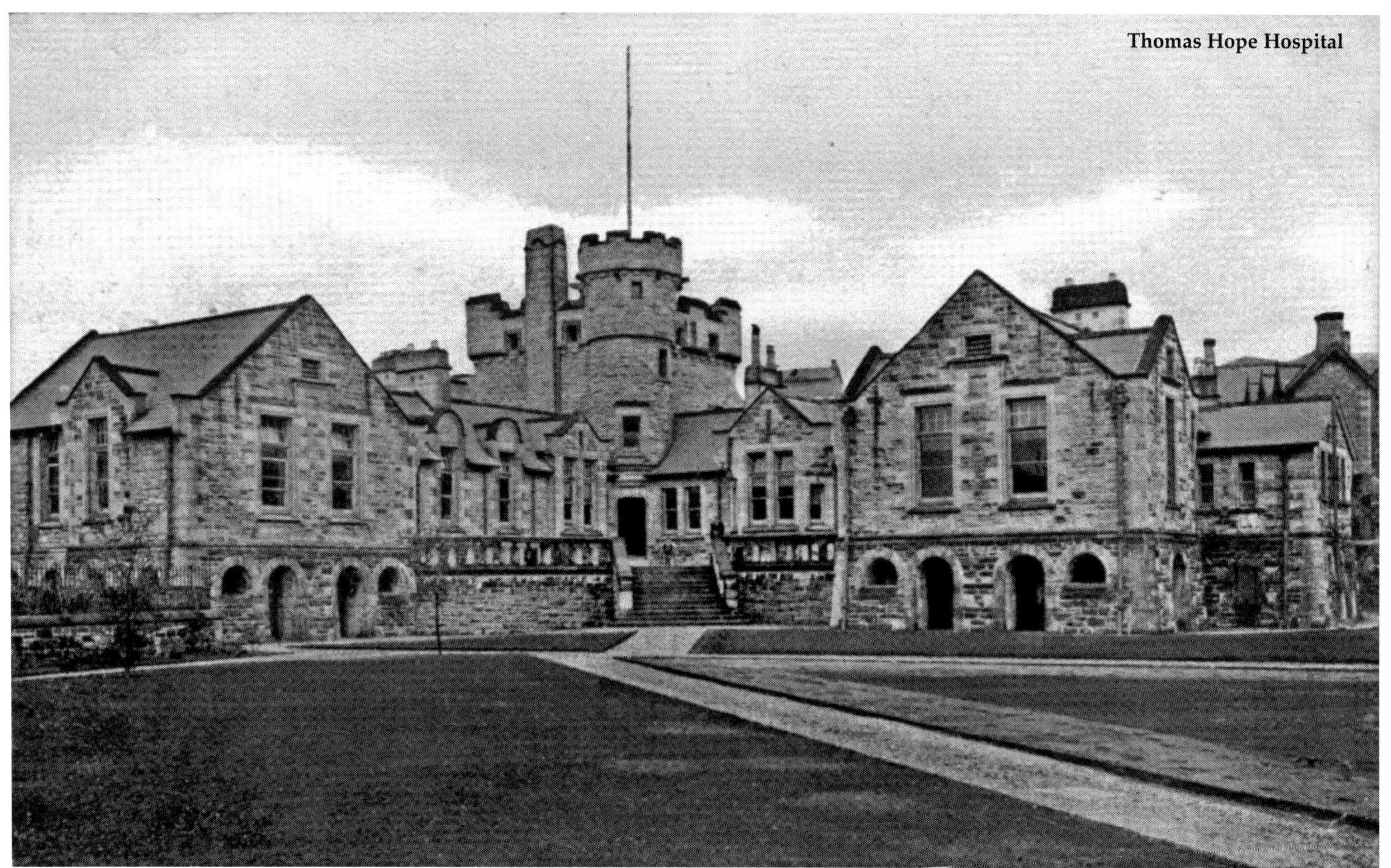


Thomas Hope Hospital in Langholm was established with a £100,000 endowment from Thomas Hope, a native of Langholm, who became a grocery magnate in the USA. It was not to be very large, but was stipulated to be of good architectural character. Abounding in personality, indeed weighing on the side of eccentricity, this substantially built cottage hospital designed by John Henry Townsend Wodd of London is of Jacobean style, and the bold central tower, octagonal operating theatre and mortuary, and elaborate ironwork gates are some of its notable features. It opened in 1897, and in 1973 accommodated a surprisingly small number of 14 beds. It is now a 12 bed community hospital.

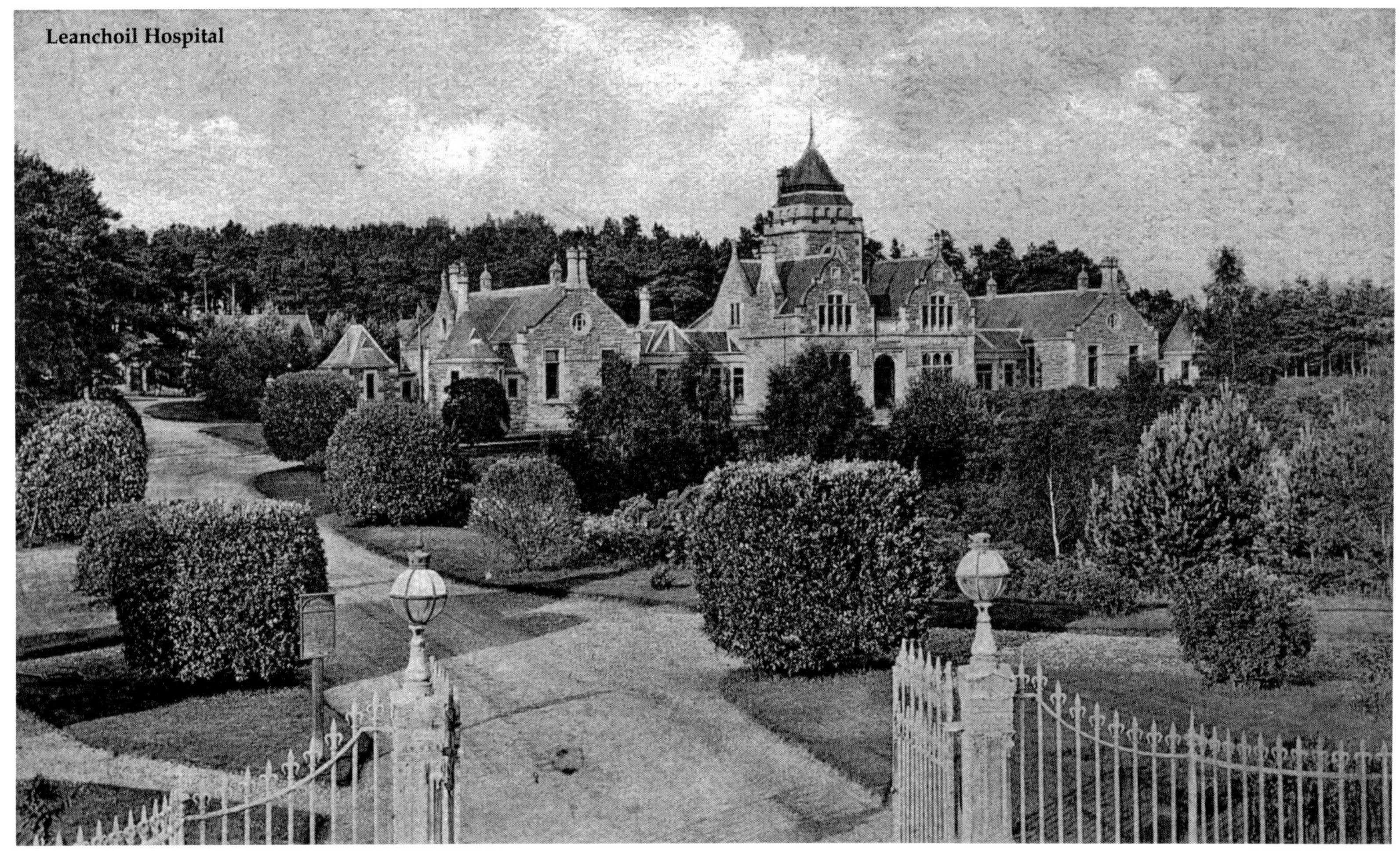
Leanchoil Hospital

Endowed by Sir Donald Smith, later Lord Strathcona, a native of Forres who made his fortune in Canada and famously drove in the last spike of the Canadian Pacific Railway at Craigellachie, this hospital opened in 1892; he left a further bequest of £10,000 to the hospital on his death in 1914. The name Leanchoil came from Smith's mother's birthplace Leth na Kyle near Abernethy. With its blend of Baronial (for the WCs) and Jacobean features and a central square tower, the hospital designed by John Rhind of Inverness has great architectural charm. The wards were heated by ventilating stoves especially designed for the building, and the floors were laid with wax-polished Canadian maple. It was extended in 1938, 1940 and the 1960s, and had 50 general and maternity beds in 1973. The maternity unit closed in 1996, and it now functions as a 9 bed community hospital.

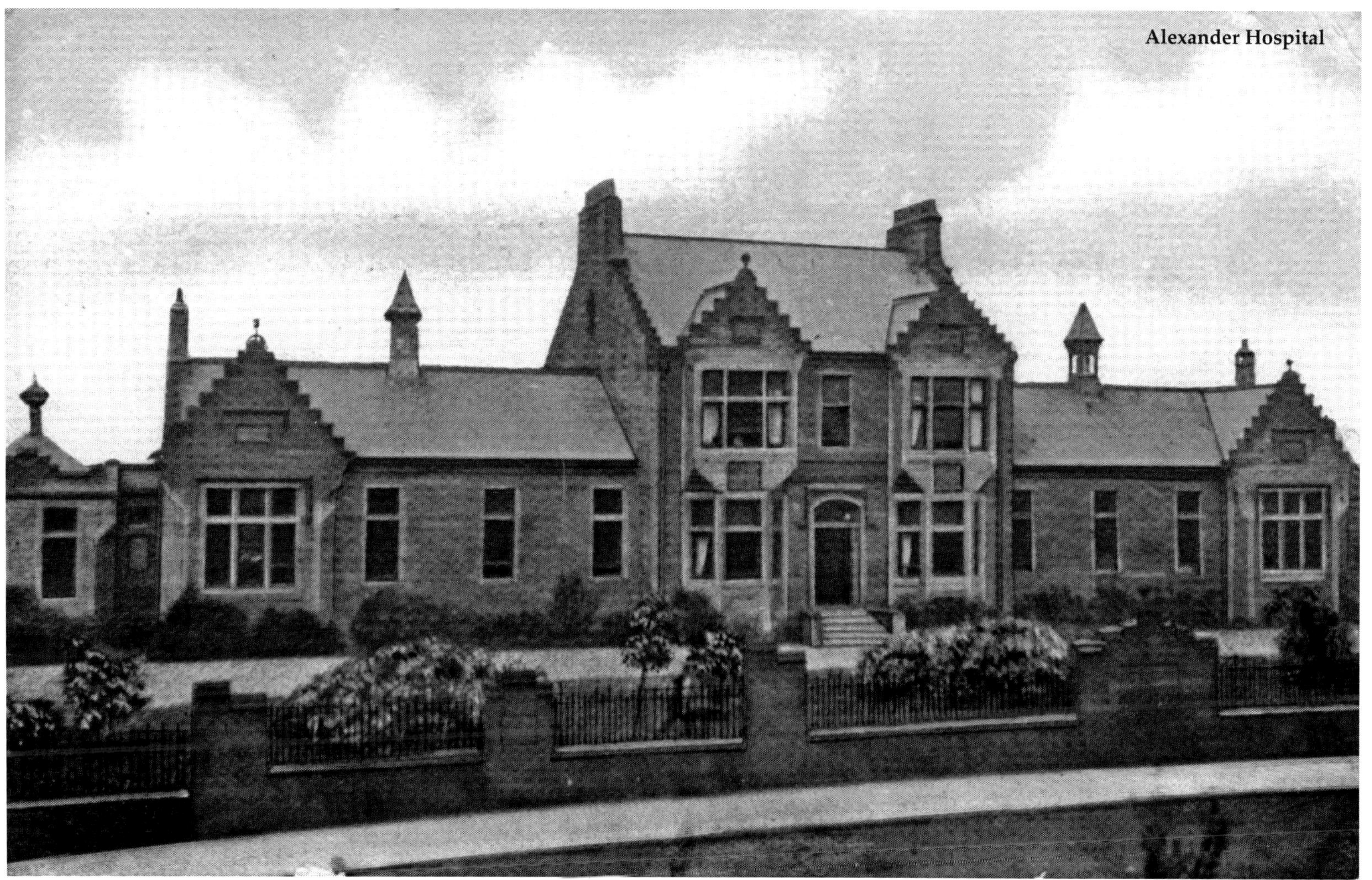

Alexander Hospital

Provost John Alexander of Coatbridge bequested £30,000 for a cottage hospital to be named after him, built of red sandstone in the Scottish Baronial style. It opened for surgical and non-infectious cases in 1899 with 20 beds, and x-ray, ward, theatre, and general practitioner maternity extensions were added over the years so that there were 32 beds in wartime and 63 general and maternity beds by 1973. Ward closure came in 1978 with conversion to the Alexander Resource Centre, a hub for local people and their communities. Final closure came in 2005, and demolition after a fire in 2009.

# Voluntary hospitals – Cottage hospitals

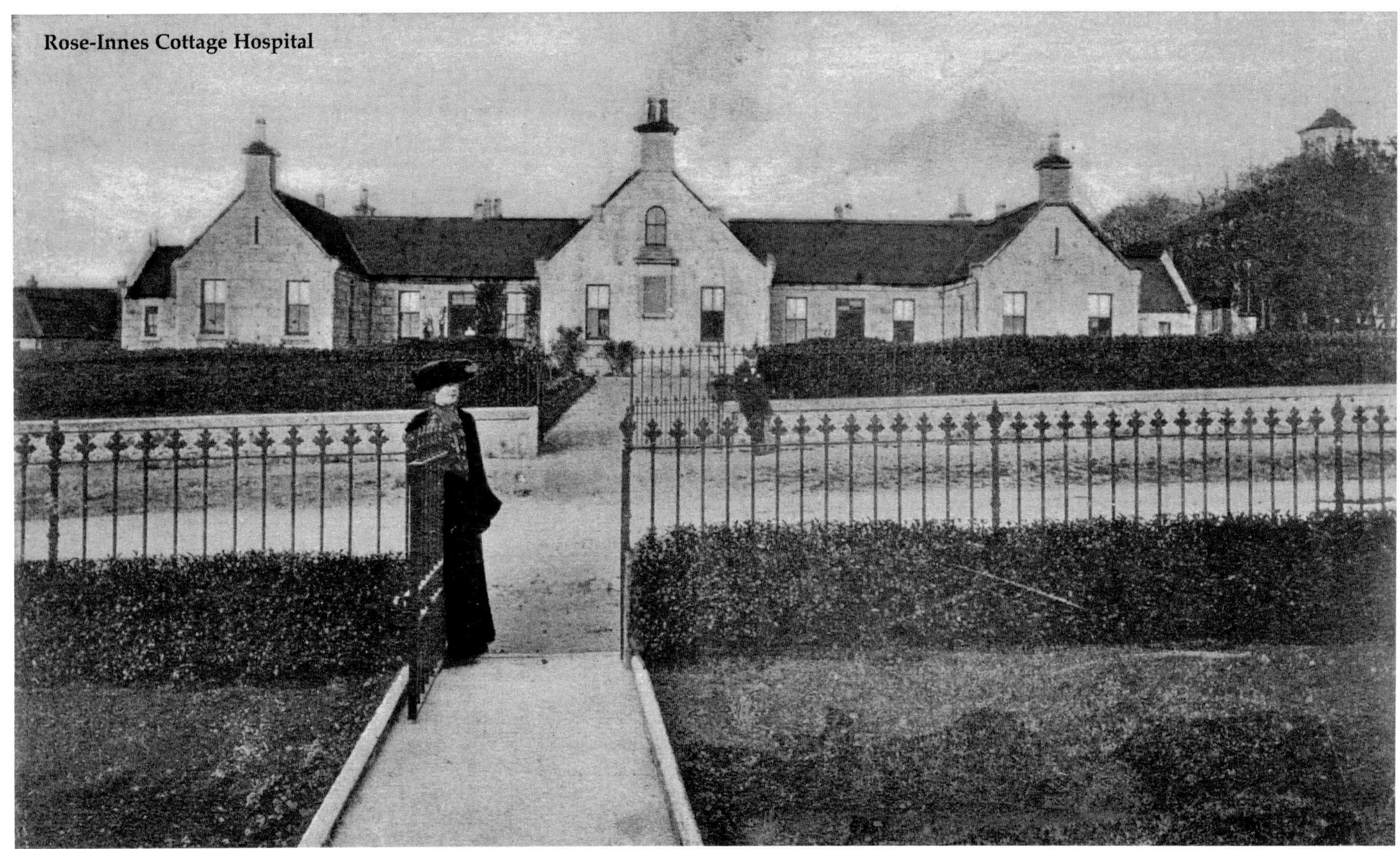

Rose-Innes Cottage Hospital

The Rose-Innes Cottage Hospital in Aberchirder was endowed by Miss Rose-Innes of Netherdale, opening in 1894. Fever cases were admitted initially, although they could be isolated if necessary by means of glass screens. By wartime it had 18 beds for medical, chronic sick, minor surgical and occasional maternity cases, and three huts for tuberculous patients. A maternity ward was added in 1950, but the hospital closed in 1958 and reopened as an old people's home the following year.

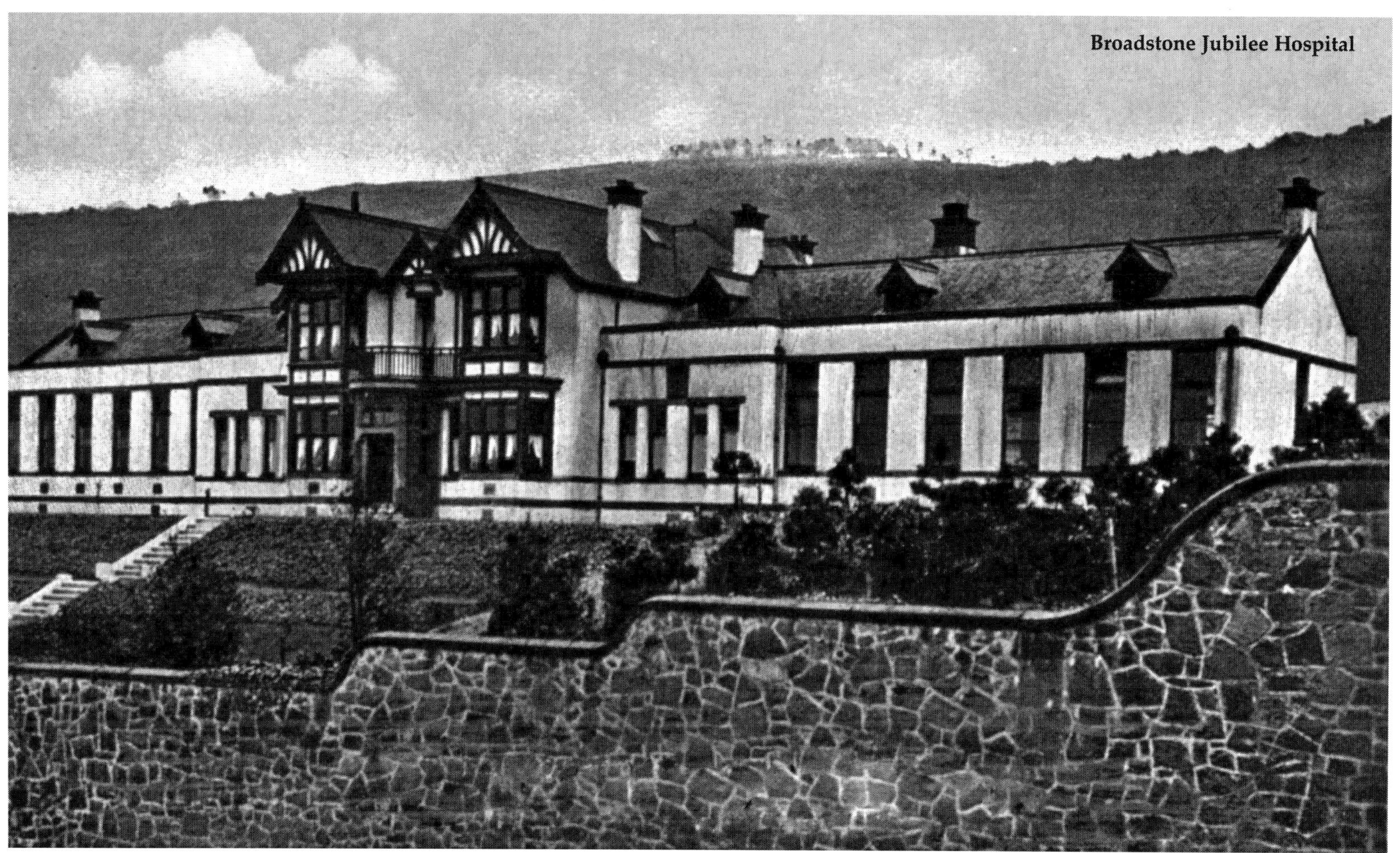

Broadstone Jubilee Hospital

Broadstone Jubilee Hospital opened in 1907 with 24 beds and a modern operating theatre. It was a gift to the people of Port Glasgow from John and Helen Birkmyre on the occasion of their golden wedding anniversary, and was intended to be a voluntary general surgical hospital for locals, particularly for the treatment of accidents which occurred in the local shipbuilding industry. The white-painted buildings must have shone out over the neighbourhood like a beacon of health. Patients were expected to contribute in other ways than merely financial, for example attending other patients, help with housework, needlework or gardening. The hospital is no longer standing; services were moved in 1979 to Inverclyde Royal Hospital in Greenock, and in its place is a sheltered housing accommodation complex for the elderly.

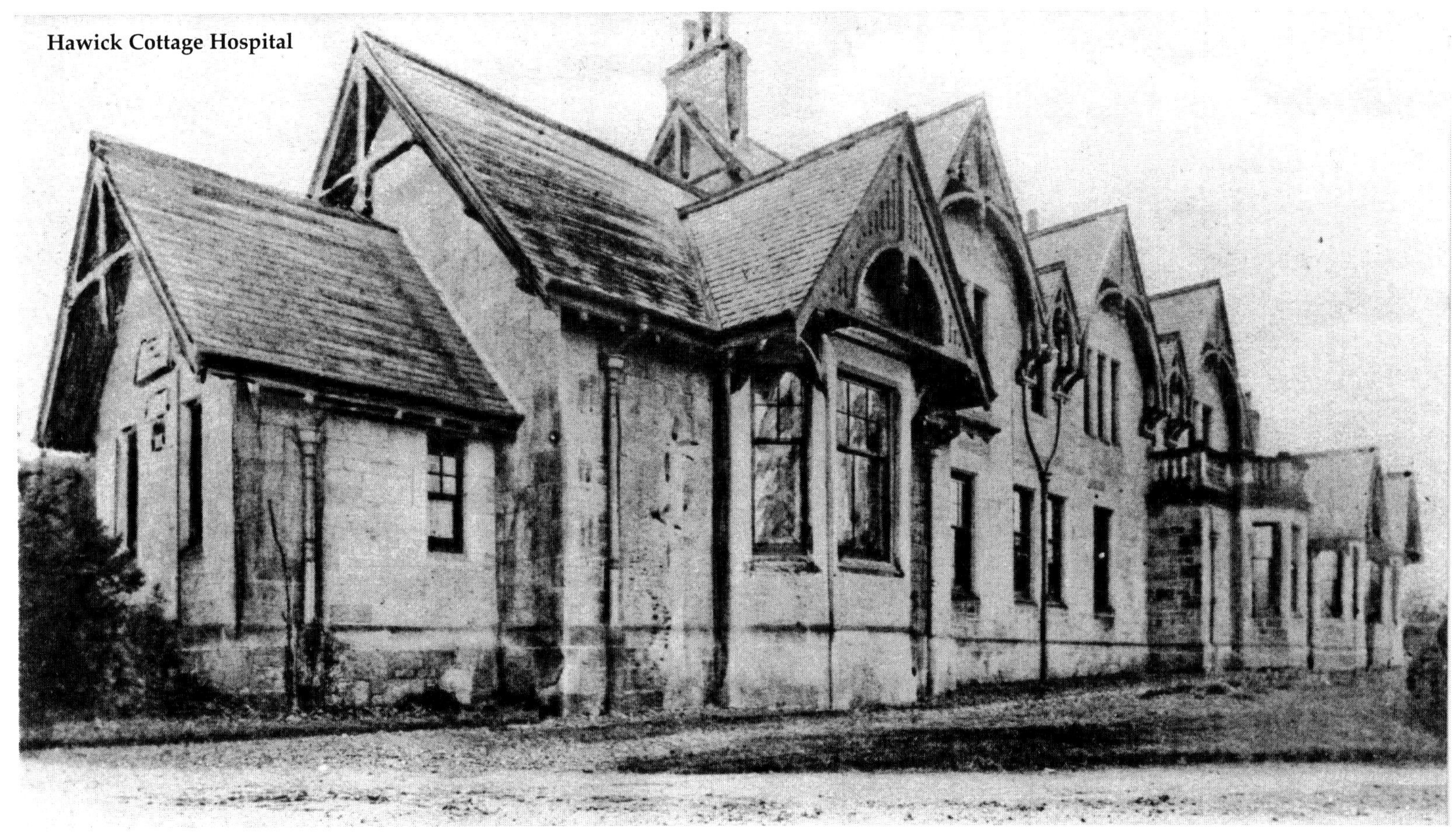


Hawick Cottage Hospital was funded by public subscription and a bazaar, this 30 bed purpose-built hospital in a good site on high ground opened in 1885. Designed by John McLachlan from Edinburgh, it was built in a cottage style with Arts and Crafts detailing such as decorative timber barge boarding, and additions in 1924 and 1933 were sympathetic and formed a cohesive whole. Between the wars Hawick admitted mostly surgical cases like other cottage hospitals, quite unlike the present day where the emphasis is on palliative medicine, rehabilitation and respite care. A new community hospital provides 24 beds and the old hospital was sold in 2012 for housing.

## Randolph Wemyss Memorial Hospital

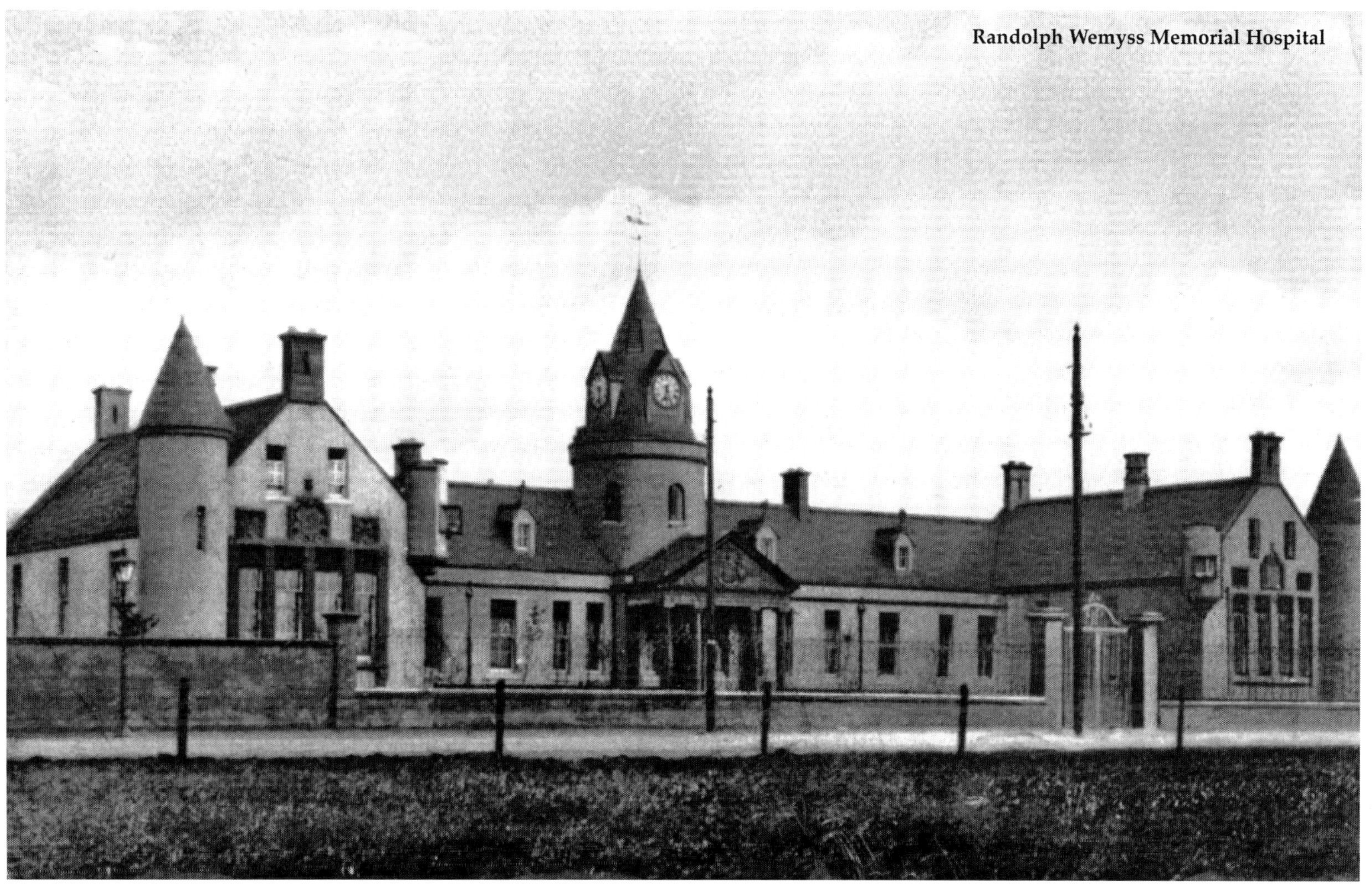

Commissioned by Randolph Wemyss' widow Lady Eva Wemyss as a memorial to her husband, this Scots Renaissance style hospital opened in 1909, built of white harl and red sandstone with a striking clock tower. There is said to have been a tunnel for injured miners linking the hospital to the nearby Wellesley Colliery which was owned by the Wemyss Coal Company from 1905 until its closure in 1967. The hospital was extended in the 1960s, and upgraded in 2008 to a 16 bed community hospital.

# Infectious disease (fever) hospitals

**Aboyne Hospital**

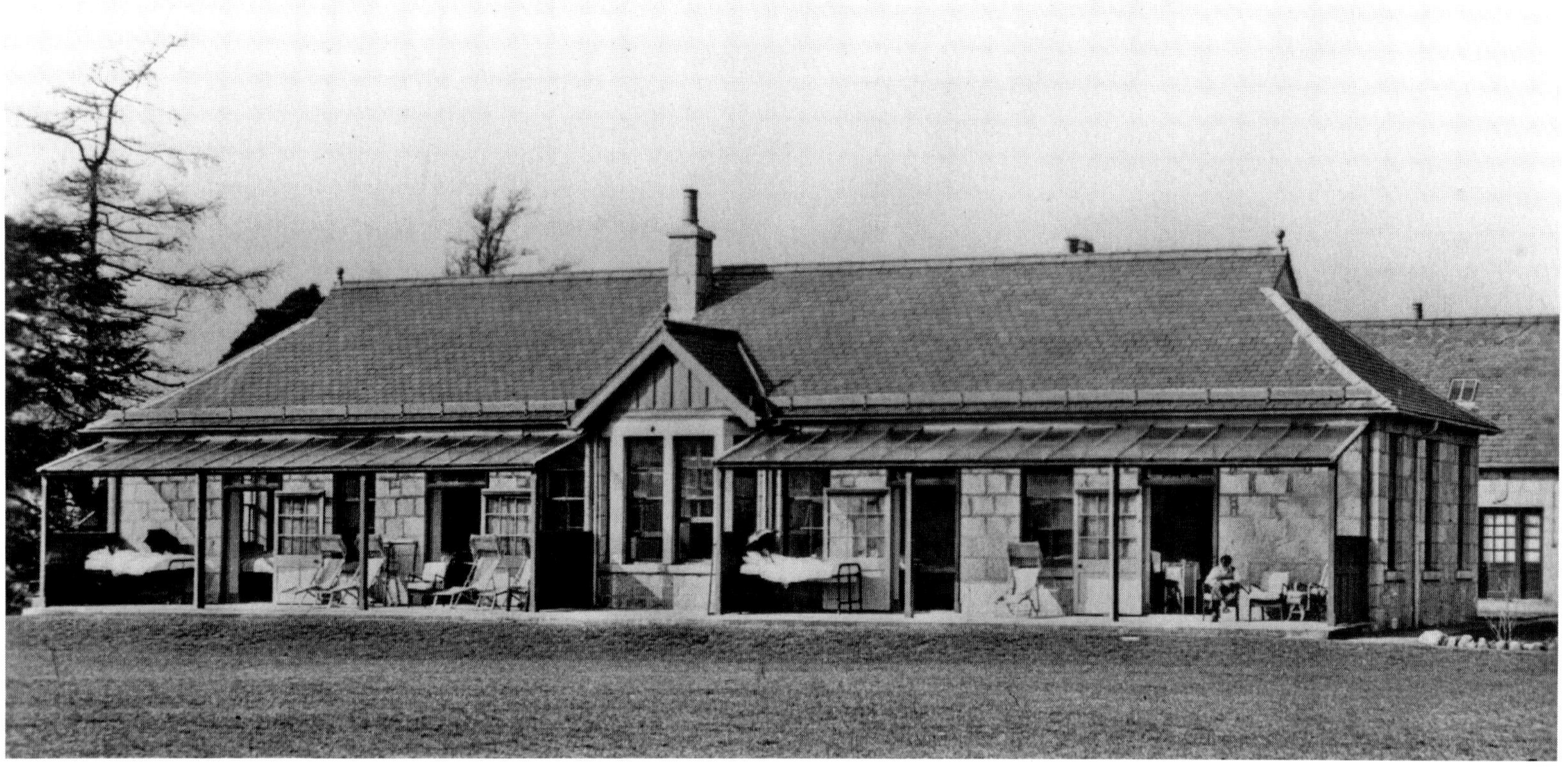

Aboyne Hospital opened in 1898 as an infectious diseases hospital, 9 years after the Public Health Act came into force which made local authorities responsible for providing such accommodation. This delay was due to difficulty in finding an appropriate site, and also local inhabitant opposition due to concerns about the hospital affecting property valuation and contamination of the water supply; there was even a whip-round for Deeside District Council to build elsewhere, but the £1,000 inducement came too late as building had already begun. The hospital was extended to 36 beds in the 1920s, and the following decade was the hospital's busiest years due to closure of Ballater and Braemar's fever hospitals, admitting a wider range of diseases such as whooping cough, chickenpox and erysipelas in addition to the usual scarlet fever and diphtheria of earlier years. Note how the beds have been brought out into the fresh air in this photograph. The hospital changed function in the NHS to 24 mainly long-stay geriatric beds by 1973, and is now a 17 bed community hospital.

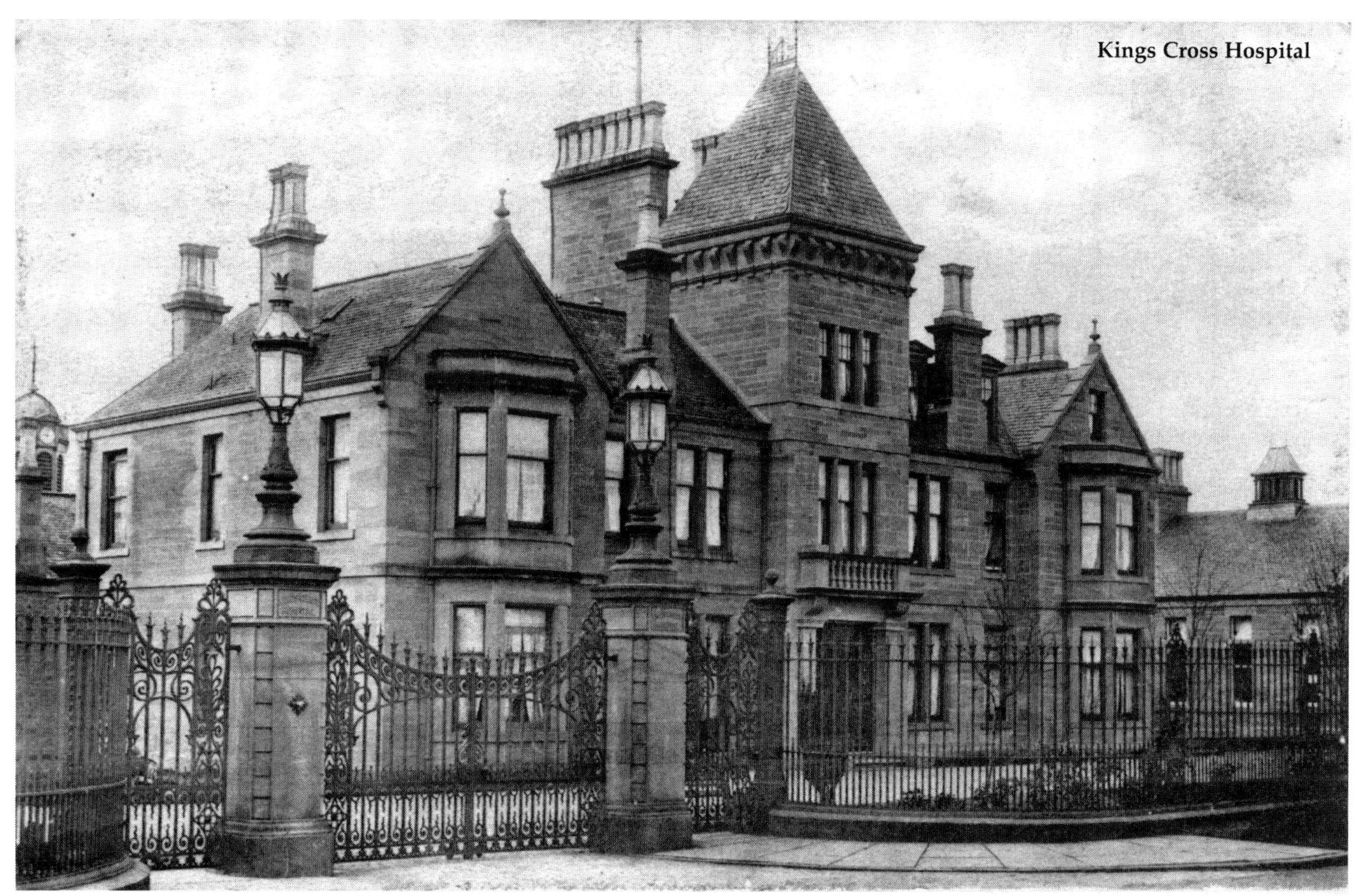

Kings Cross Hospital

Dundee Town Council acquired an isolated tenement for cholera which was well used in an 1832 epidemic, but then sold it off so that when a further 1849 cholera outbreak hit the town it was left to the Royal Infirmary to cope, as it had to do for numerous other epidemics before and since, infectious diseases at times occupying up to 85% of available beds. The Town Council dabbled with temporary structures in 1867 at Lochee for typhus and smallpox and another building at Clepington Road for scarlet fever, but despite promptings from the Royal Infirmary, it took until 1890 for Dundee to finally build Kings Cross Hospital, a proper infectious diseases hospital. This gradually enlarged until it had 250 beds by wartime. A new isolation unit based on a Swedish prototype opened in 1964 and Kings Cross later housed a chest unit, but most services moved to Ninewells Hospital in the 1990s. The administration block in the illustration shows cast iron gates, gateposts and railings of a particularly high quality, made by Walter MacFarlane's Saracen Foundry in Glasgow.

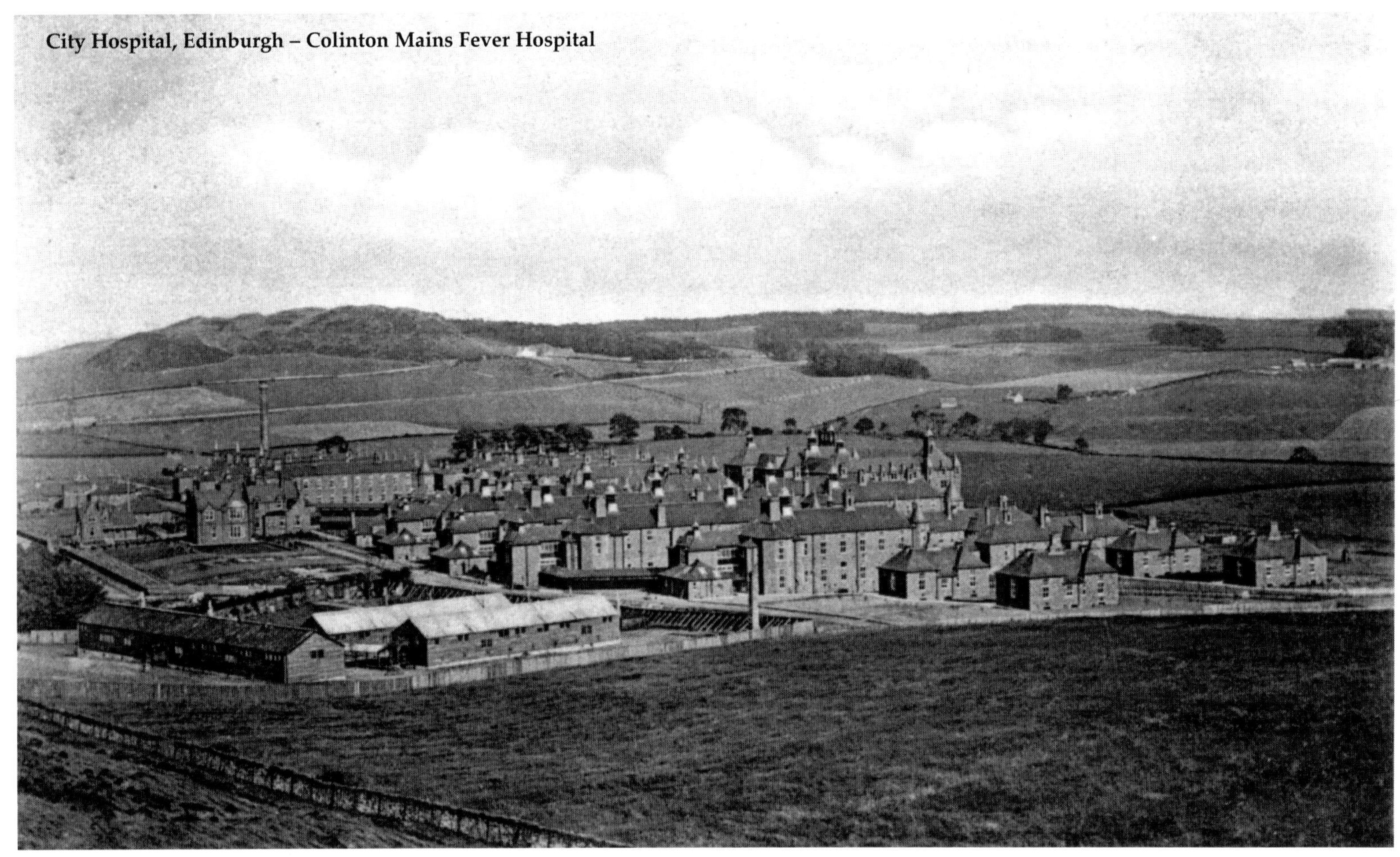

## City Hospital, Edinburgh – Colinton Mains Fever Hospital

Colinton Mains Fever Hospital had its origins in city poorhouses and part of the old Edinburgh Royal Infirmary known as the City Fever Hospital, this 779 bed hospital for infectious diseases opened in 1903 at Colinton Mains in southwest Edinburgh. Initially there were two ranks of ward pavilions ranged around a central administrative building; constructed of red sandstone, these large complexes were relatively isolated when first built. Accommodation was added for tuberculosis patients in 1913, including revolving shelters which let patients receive the basic treatments before antibiotics of rest in bed, fresh air and sunshine, at least on sunny days. By the 1960s the hospital was also treating tropical and chest disease, thoracic surgery and otolaryngology, and there were 573 beds in 1973. Closure came in 2002, with patients moving to the new Royal Infirmary. The hospital was redeveloped for housing.

## Gateside Infectious Diseases Hospital

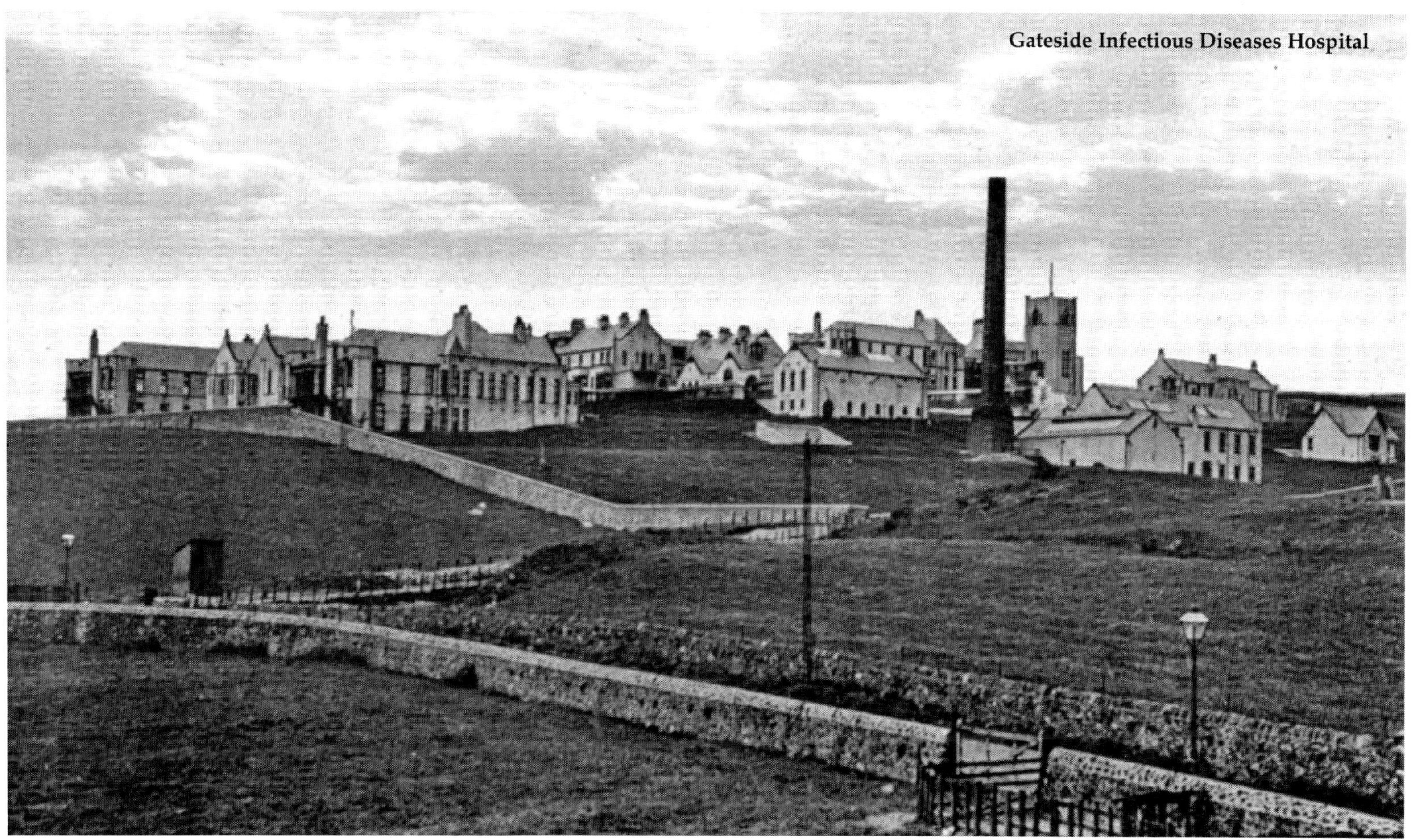

Prior to the Gateside Infectious Diseases Hospital, fever cases were admitted to Greenock Infirmary, and there was a separate smallpox hospital in the town. Opened in 1908 as a combination hospital with 104 infectious diseases and 20 tuberculosis beds, this well-planned hospital at Gateside occupied ten acres of high ground in isolation well outside the town. As the original name of Greenock and District Combination Hospital implies, representatives from the corporations of Greenock, Gourock, Port Glasgow and from Renfrew County Council jointly managed it. A novel feature was that the ward ends were circular rather than square and all internal angles and corners were rounded, all to help with the cleaning. Its function changed after the Second World War to treat general medical, orthopaedic and paediatric patients, and there were 140 beds by 1973. It closed in 1979, superseded by Inverclyde Hospital, and was subsequently demolished for housing.

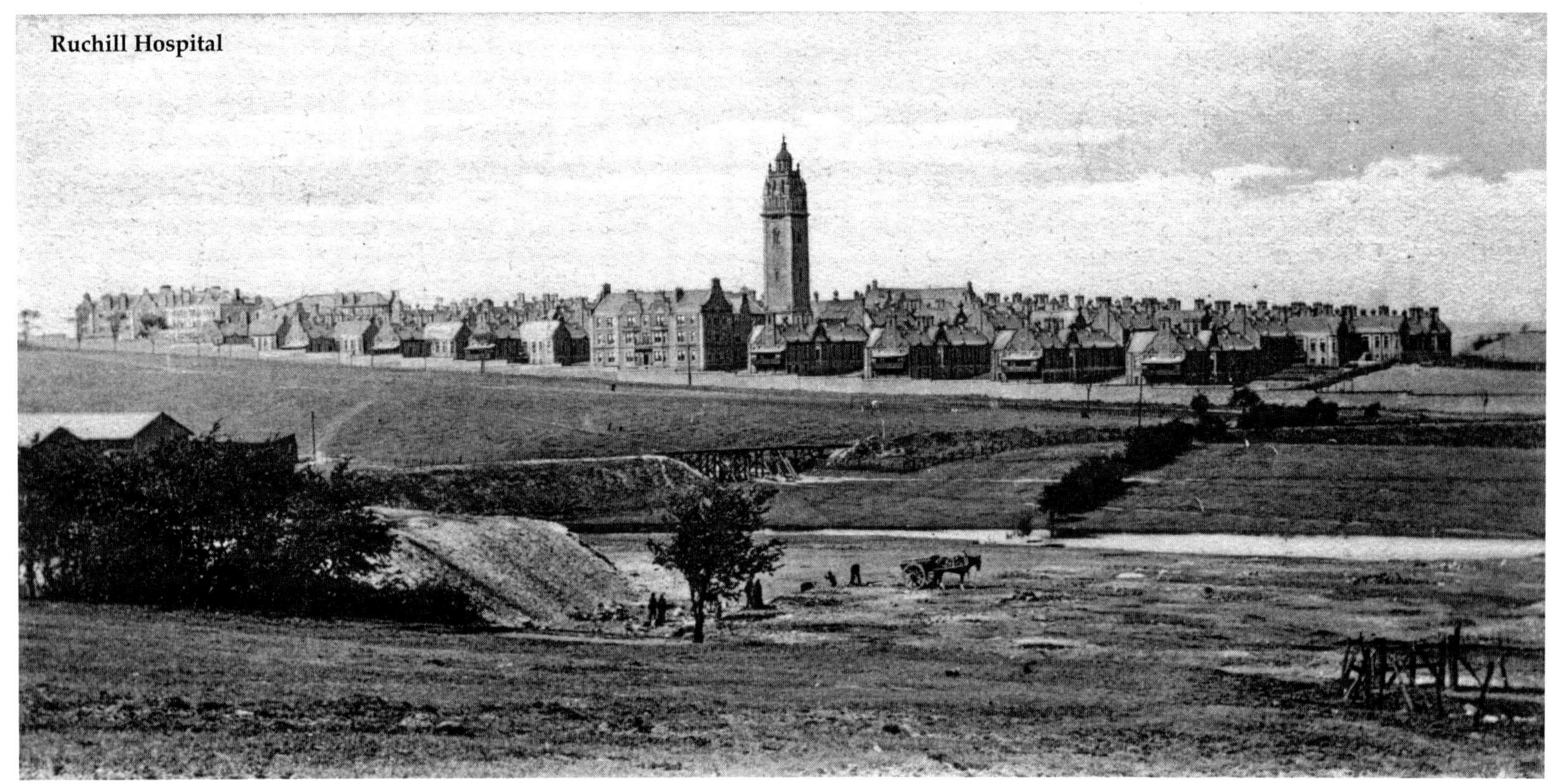

Ruchill Hospital

Situated in an industrial district, Ruchill opened in 1900 as Glasgow's second infectious diseases hospital to help relieve Belvidere Hospital's cramped conditions. The quantity of buildings on the site gave the whole the resemblance of a village. Initially housing 440 beds, pavilions for 272 tuberculosis patients followed in 1915. It incorporated all the modern developments in ventilation and sanitary facilities; its hilltop site gave problems in providing an adequate water supply, necessitating an impressive Flemish water tower which formed a distinctive landmark. Bed complement rose to 1,000 in 1948, but dropped to 280 in 1990 by which time it had been converted into mainly geriatric, psychiatric and young chronic sick (mainly catastrophic brain damage) care. In the 1980s it treated many sexually transmitted diseases and was the primary hospital in Glasgow to deal with cases of HIV, the cause of AIDS which came to prominence at that time. Closure of the hospital came in 1998 and it was sold to Scottish Enterprise.

# Sanatoria

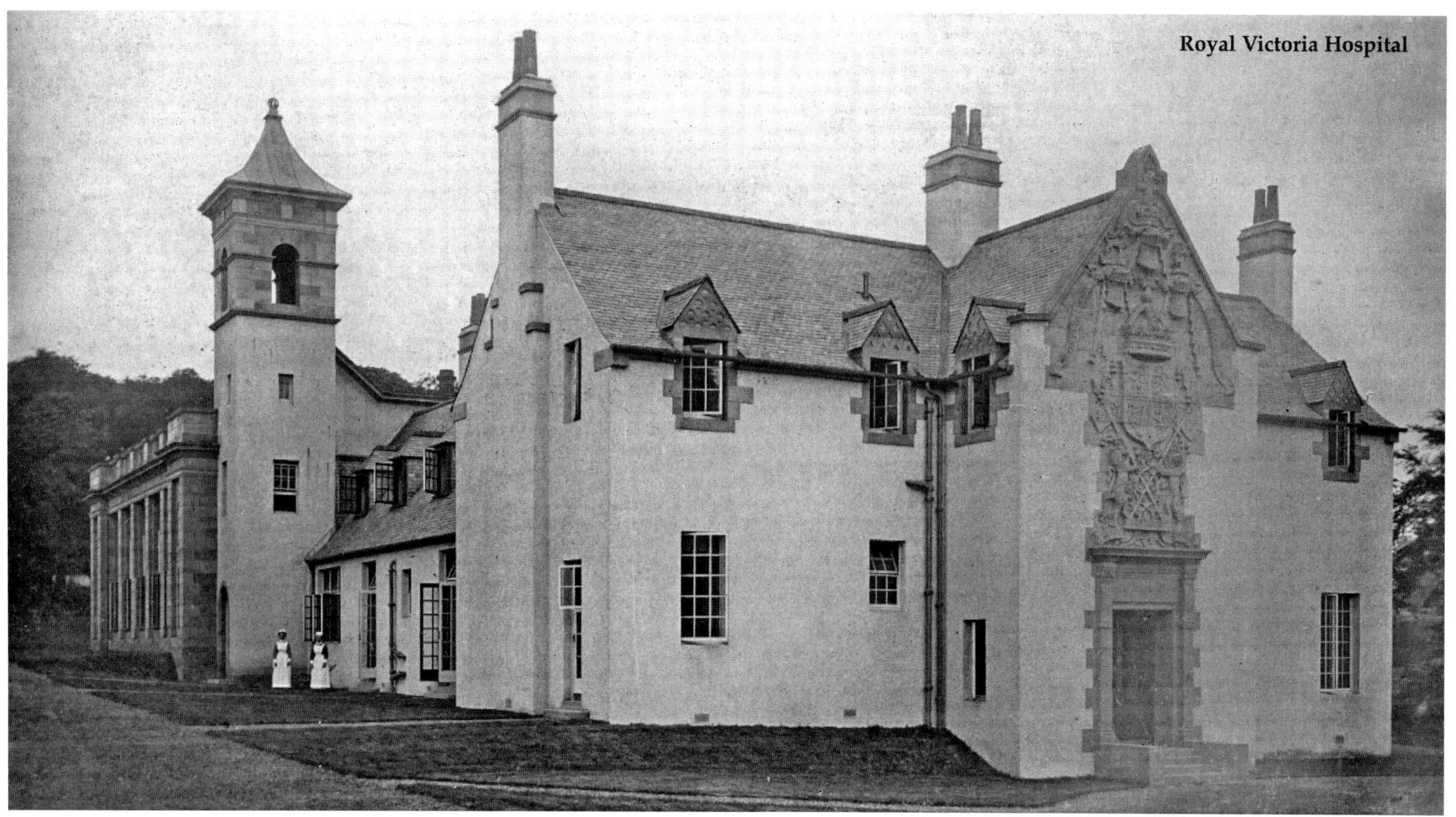

**Royal Victoria Hospital**

Royal Victoria Hospital's 1887 origin was in Dr Robert Philip's Victoria Dispensary for Consumption and Diseases of the Chest in Edinburgh, which was the first tuberculosis clinic in the world. Craigleith House followed in 1894 as a 12 bed sanatorium for more advanced cases, and Royal Patronage was granted in 1904. Philip's pioneering approach, the 'Edinburgh Scheme', lay in the combination of isolation from family and friends, sunshine with sun houses, fresh air including continuous open windows, mild exercise, education by leaflets and follow-up of contacts. By wartime there were 76 beds, housed in so-called butterfly wards due to their shape. With decline in tuberculosis in the 1950s, the hospital converted to a 247 bed geriatric unit, which relocated to the Western General Hospital in 2012. The administration building shown here has a large ornate Royal Coat of Arms above the front entrance, inscribed in Latin 'God and My Right, Who Shall Separate Us, No-one Harms Me with Impunity'.

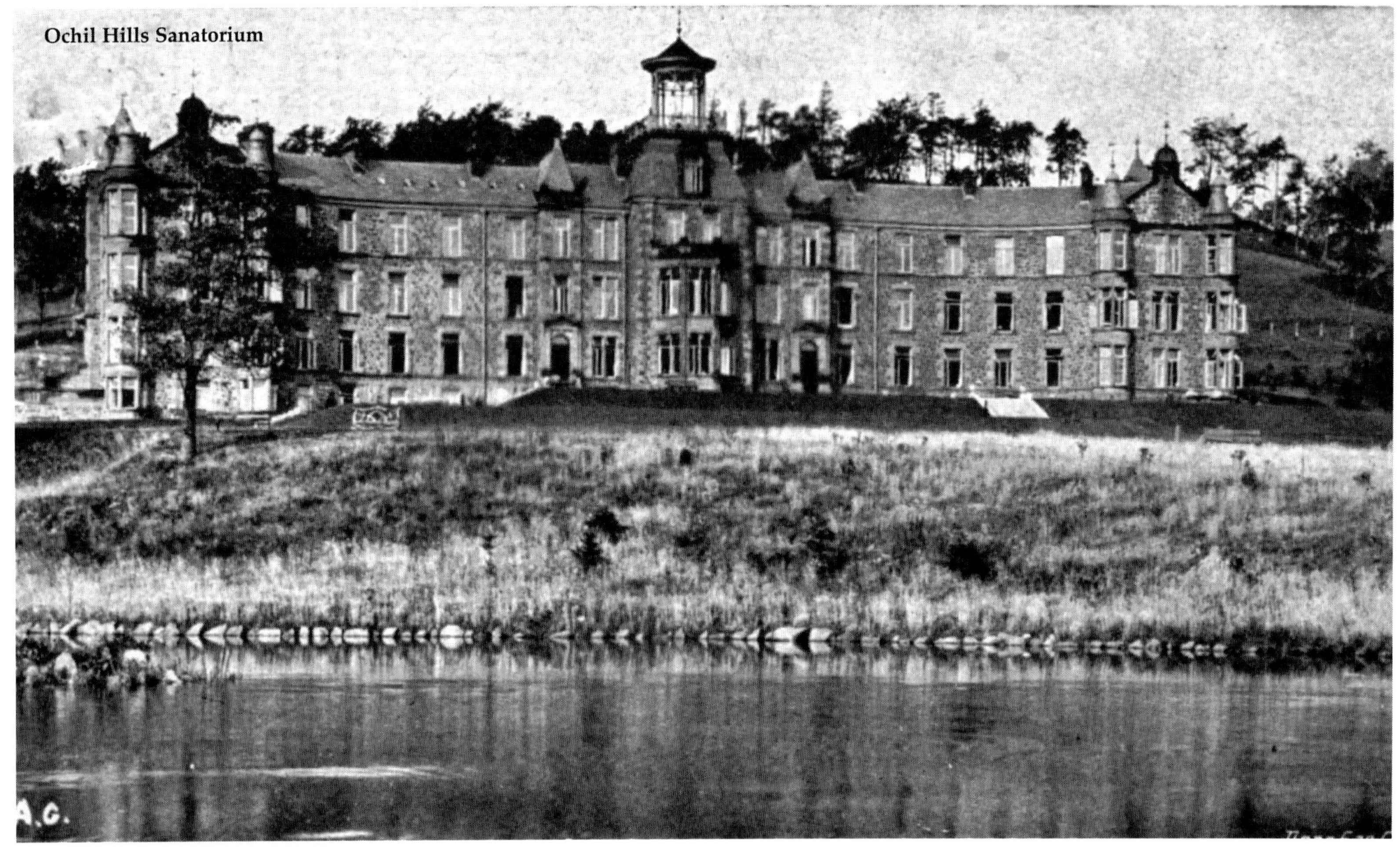


**Ochil Hills Sanatorium**

This 60 bed sanatorium was built on a fine site of 450 acres overlooking Loch Leven in 1902. It catered for well-to-do (5 guineas a week) cases of pulmonary tuberculosis from Clackmannan, Stirling, Dunfermline and also some patients from Glasgow. The rationale of sanatoria was that rest, fresh air and good nutrition offered the best chance that the sufferer's immune system would 'wall off' pockets of pulmonary tuberculosis infection. A British Medical Journal article in 1900 claimed that the mortality from tuberculosis in Kinross-shire was lower than in any other part of the United Kingdom. By wartime there were 110 beds, but by 1973 the hospital had changed function to 88 convalescent beds. The hospital closed in 1987 and was demolished after a fire in 2003.

Bridge of Weir Sanatorium
ELISE HOSPITAL, ORPHAN HOMES OF SCOTLAND, BRIDGE OF WEIR.

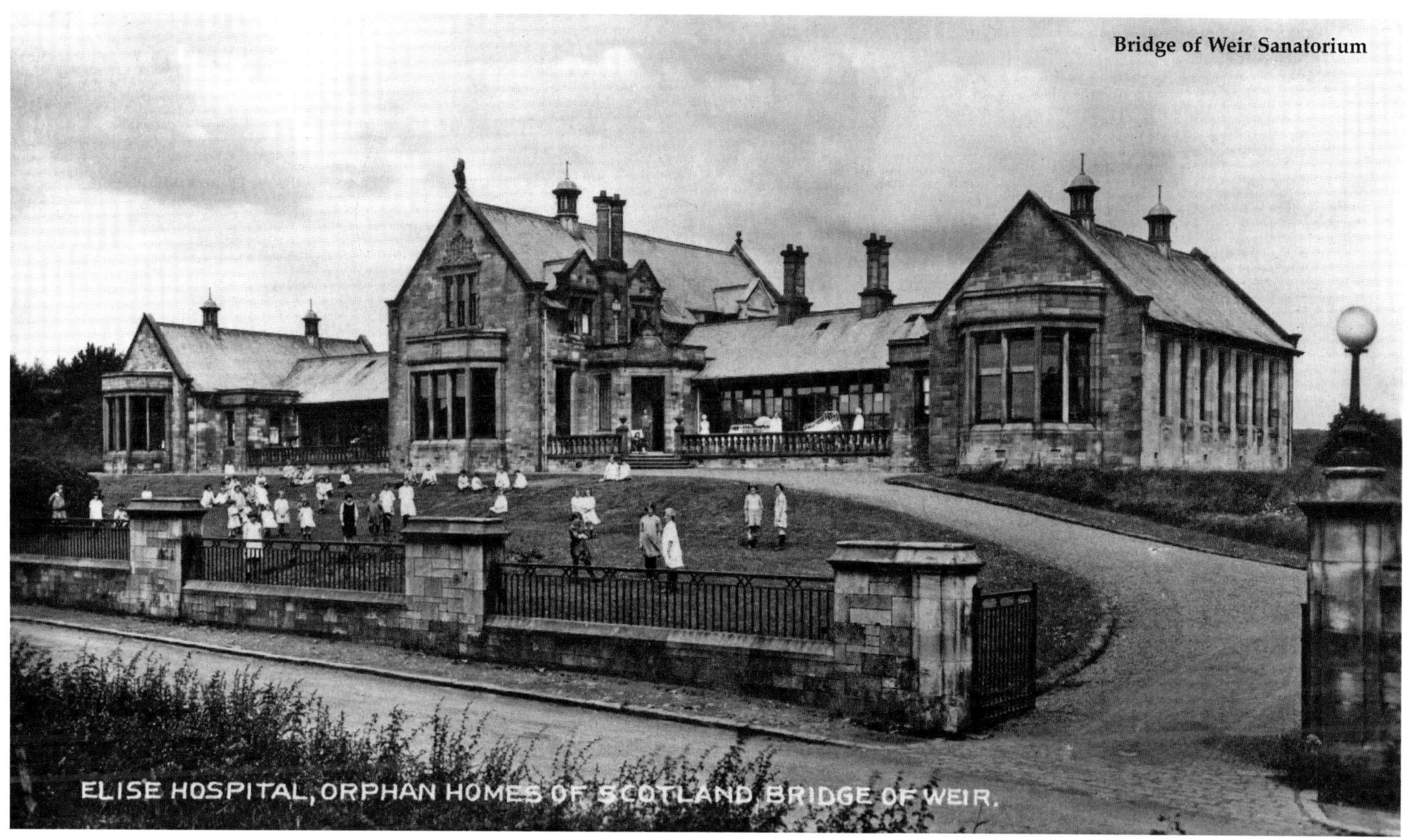

This large group of buildings which opened between 1896 and 1912 were contained within William Quarrier's orphan homes, three large red sandstone pavilion sanatoria and a colony for epileptics which was unusual for its time. There was plenty of fresh air and room for gentle exercise for the tuberculosis patients, and by wartime there were about 200 tuberculosis beds and 130 for epileptics. As the need for tuberculosis in-patient treatment diminished, conversion to geriatric and chronic sick took place and in 1973 there were 151 beds. The geriatric hospital closed in 1999 to become residential flats and the orphan homes have been converted into private housing. Hunter House was Scotland's only residential epilepsy assessment centre until this facility moved to Glasgow in 2013. Elise Hospital could accommodate 30 patients, mainly childhood infectious diseases such as measles, scarlet fever and diphtheria, and is now an old people's home.

# Hospitals for incurables

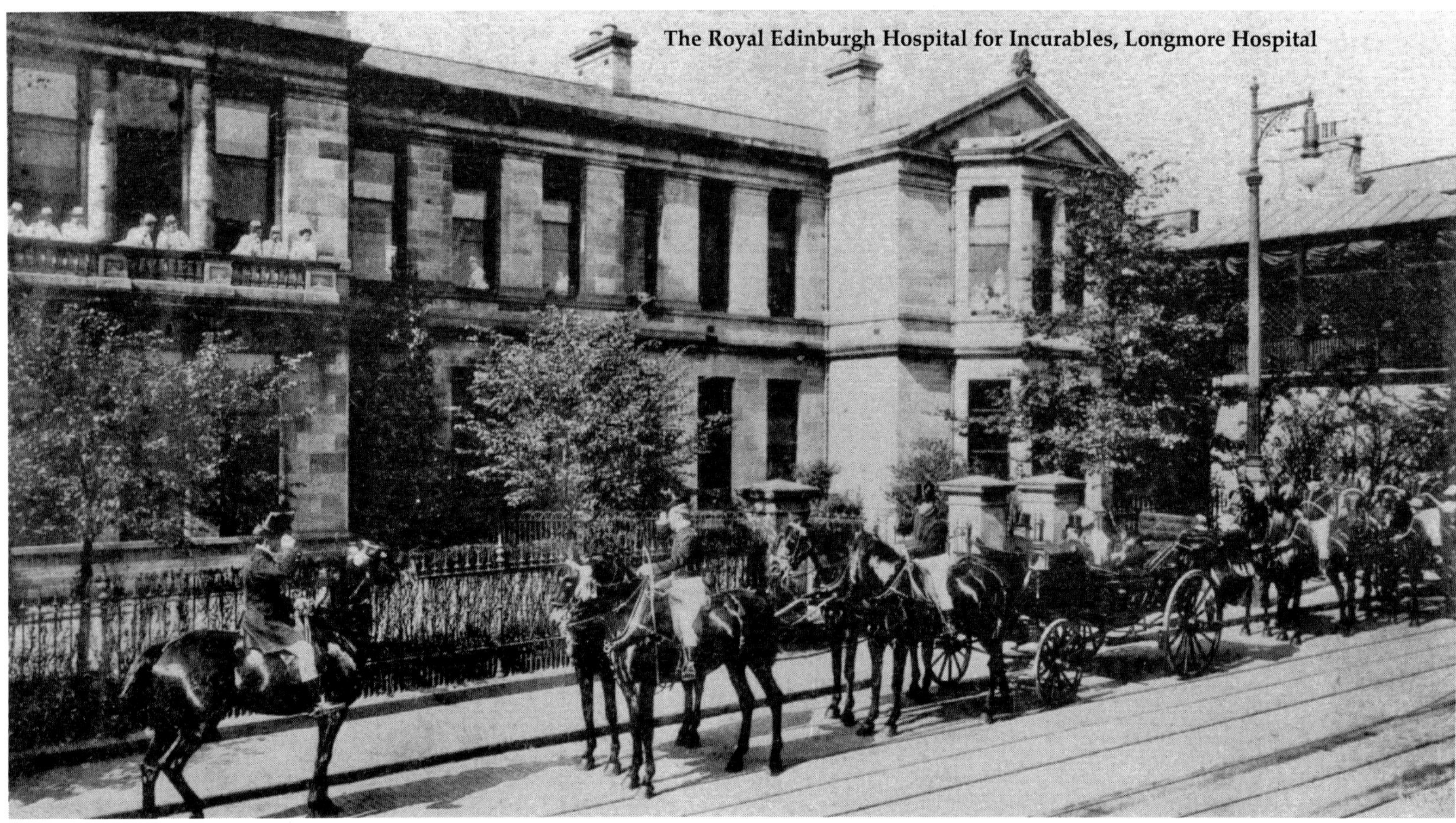

The Royal Edinburgh Hospital for Incurables, Longmore Hospital

Endowed by John Longmore to the tune of £10,000, the Edinburgh Hospital for Incurables in Newington opened in 1875 with 22 beds; the Edinburgh Association for the Relief of Incurables then purchased adjacent buildings and commissioned a new hospital to a neoclassical design by John More Dick Peddie in 1880. A new west wing in 1899 accommodated phthisical (tuberculous) patients on the ground floor and cancer patients on the upper floor. Receiving its Royal Charter in 1903, the hospital was extended five years later to include Liberton Hospital which mainly treated younger patients with incurable disease. Extensions brought the bed complement up to 150 by wartime, and in later days the hospital was responsible for breast cancer care. Longmore Hospital closed in 1991, services transferring to the Western General Hospital. The building is now headquarters for Historic Environment Scotland. The postcard likely depicts a visit from the Lord High Commissioner.

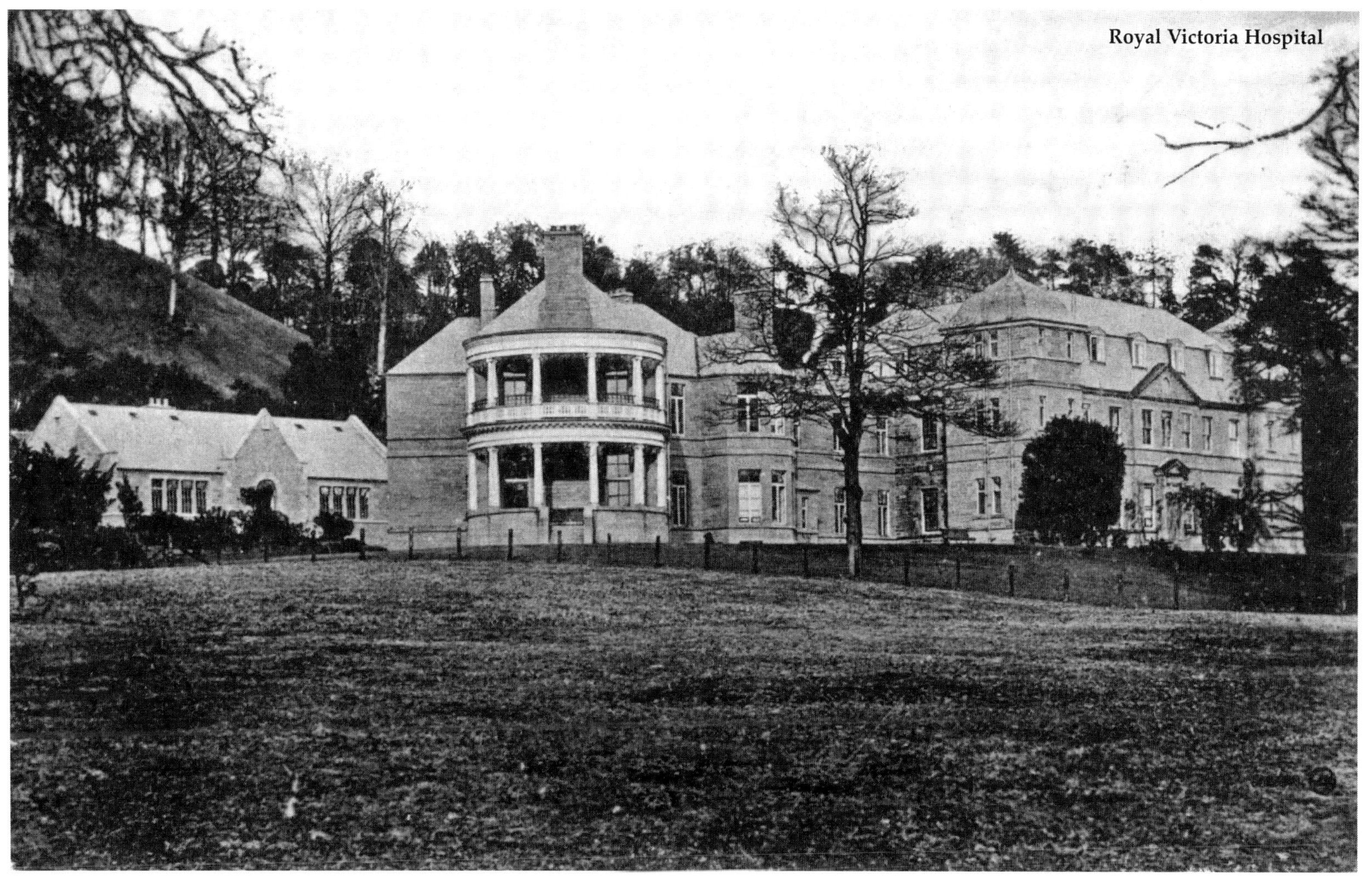


The Royal Victoria Hospital is centred on the 1760s Balgay House in the West End of Dundee which was purchased by The Society in Aid of Incurable Persons in Dundee and District to provide long-term nursing care for terminally-ill patients. It opened in 1899 to commemorate Queen Victoria's Diamond Jubilee of 1897 and a cancer wing with semicircular balconies was added in 1906, as shown here. By the Second World War there were 52 beds and in 1973 there were 138 beds for chronic disease and geriatric medicine. A centre for brain injury rehabilitation and Roxburghe House for palliative care are more recent additions.

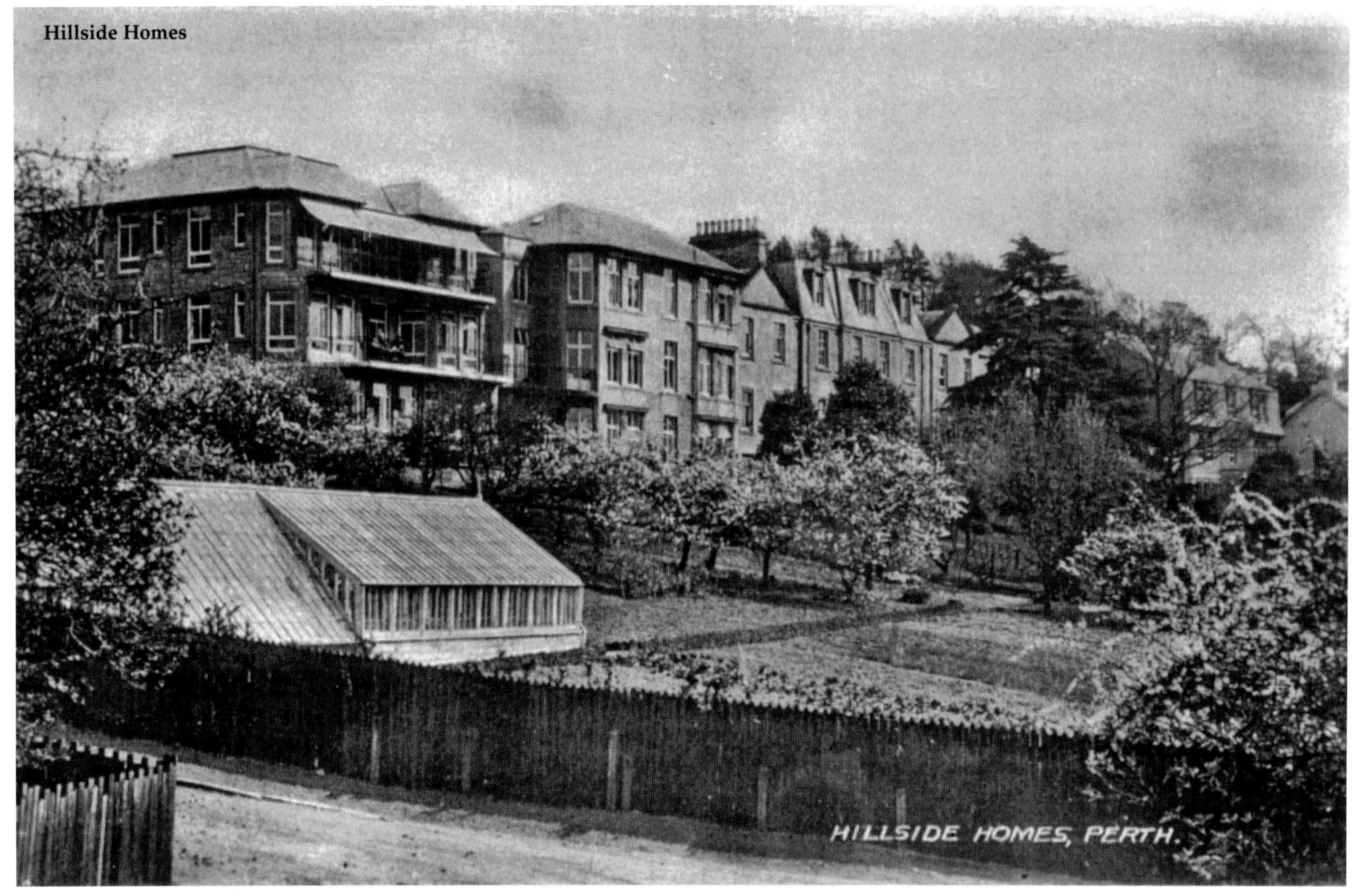


The 80 bed Hillside Homes for the chronic sick was founded in 1876 and moved to this site in 1883. Five years later a building was provided for patients with consumption, a wasting condition from pulmonary tuberculosis. In 1973, there were 100 geriatric beds (derived from Greek *geros* old age and *iatrikos* of a physician). It closed in 1997 and was demolished ten years later for housing.

# Poor Law hospitals

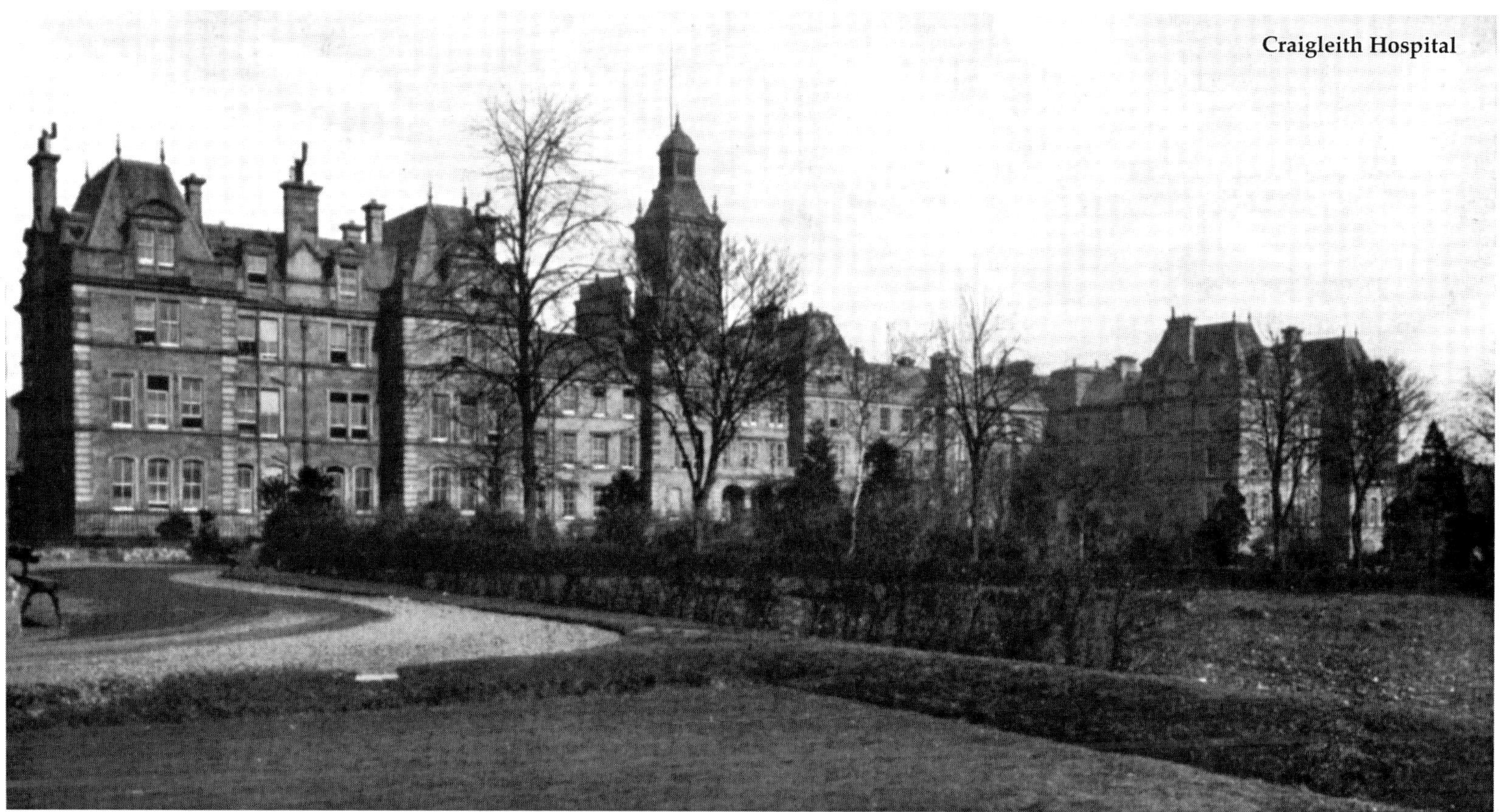

Craigleith Hospital

Built in 1868 to house the poor and destitute of the Parish of St. Cuthbert's, Craigleith Poorhouse and Hospital served the needs of the Parish's paupers until 1914 when it was taken over by the army during the First World War when it was known as the 2nd Scottish General Hospital, Craigleith was used for military casualties and had its own magazine, the *Craigleith Chronicle*. In 1931 it became known as the Western General Hospital after the Local Government Act gave management to Edinburgh Town Council, the bed complement rising from 120 to 300. In 1941, part of the hospital with 120 beds was given over to the Polish School of Medicine and became known as the Paderewski Hospital for Polish soldiers and civilians, the Paderewski fund in New York ensuring that the hospital was well-funded; it closed at the end of 1947, but plans to replicate the medical school and hospital in Poland were prevented by post-war political changes in Eastern Europe. The Western General underwent many additions in the National Health Service, and is now a 570 bed general and specialist hospital, renowned for the treatment of cancer and neurological disorders.

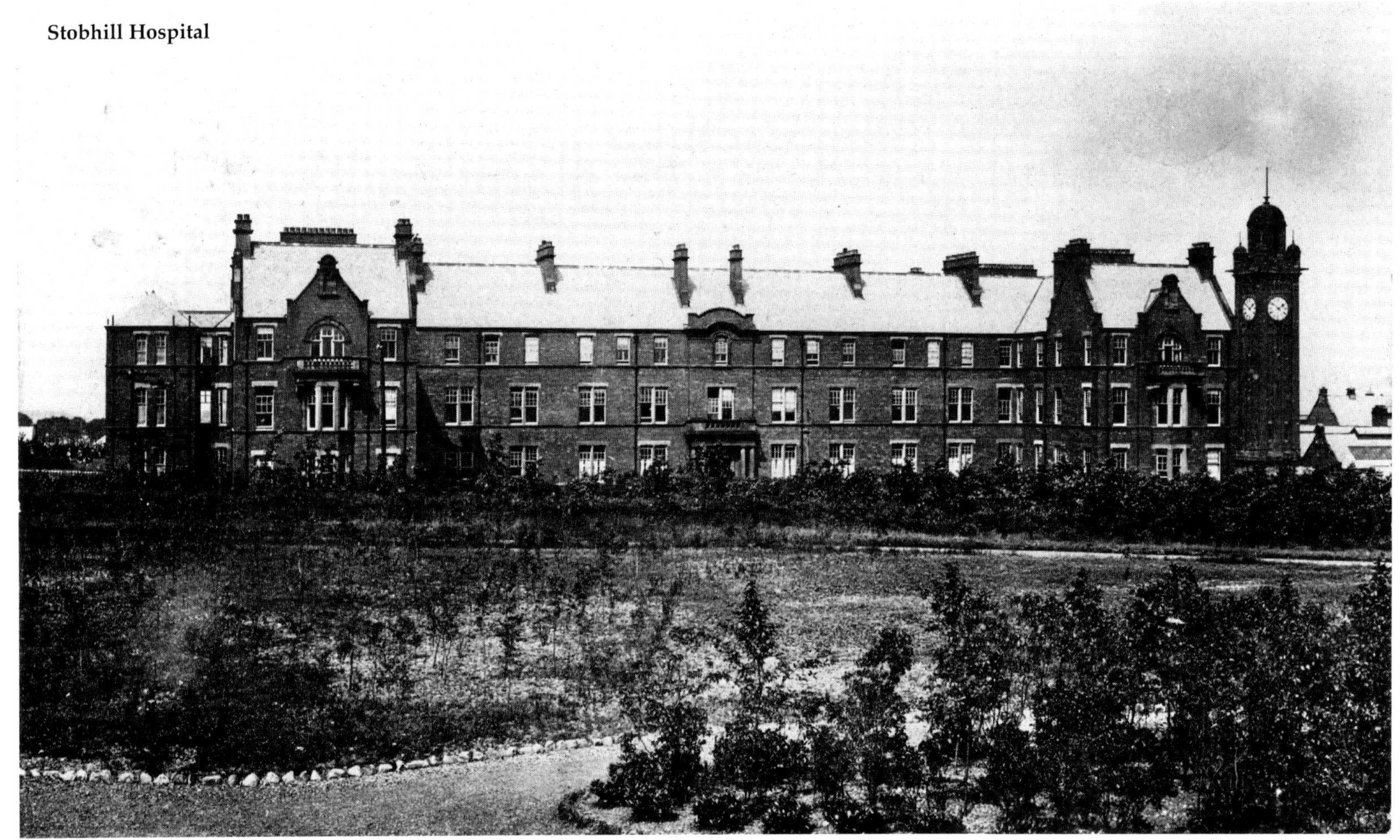

Opened in 1904 with 1,867 beds, this Poor Law hospital was built by Glasgow Parish Council. The site was dominated by a giant water tower which was mainly brick with a prominent clock and cupola. During the Second World War it became known as the 3rd and 4th Scottish General Hospitals, and was well-suited for this military role as it could handle ambulance trains at a temporary railway platform within the hospital grounds. Taken over by Glasgow Corporation in 1930 after the Local Government Act, in 1937 Stobhill became a teaching hospital, the first in Scotland outwith the voluntary sector. In 1973 there were 1,057 general and maternity beds. Stobhill is now an ambulatory care and diagnostic hospital with 185 mental health and 12 short-stay surgical beds.

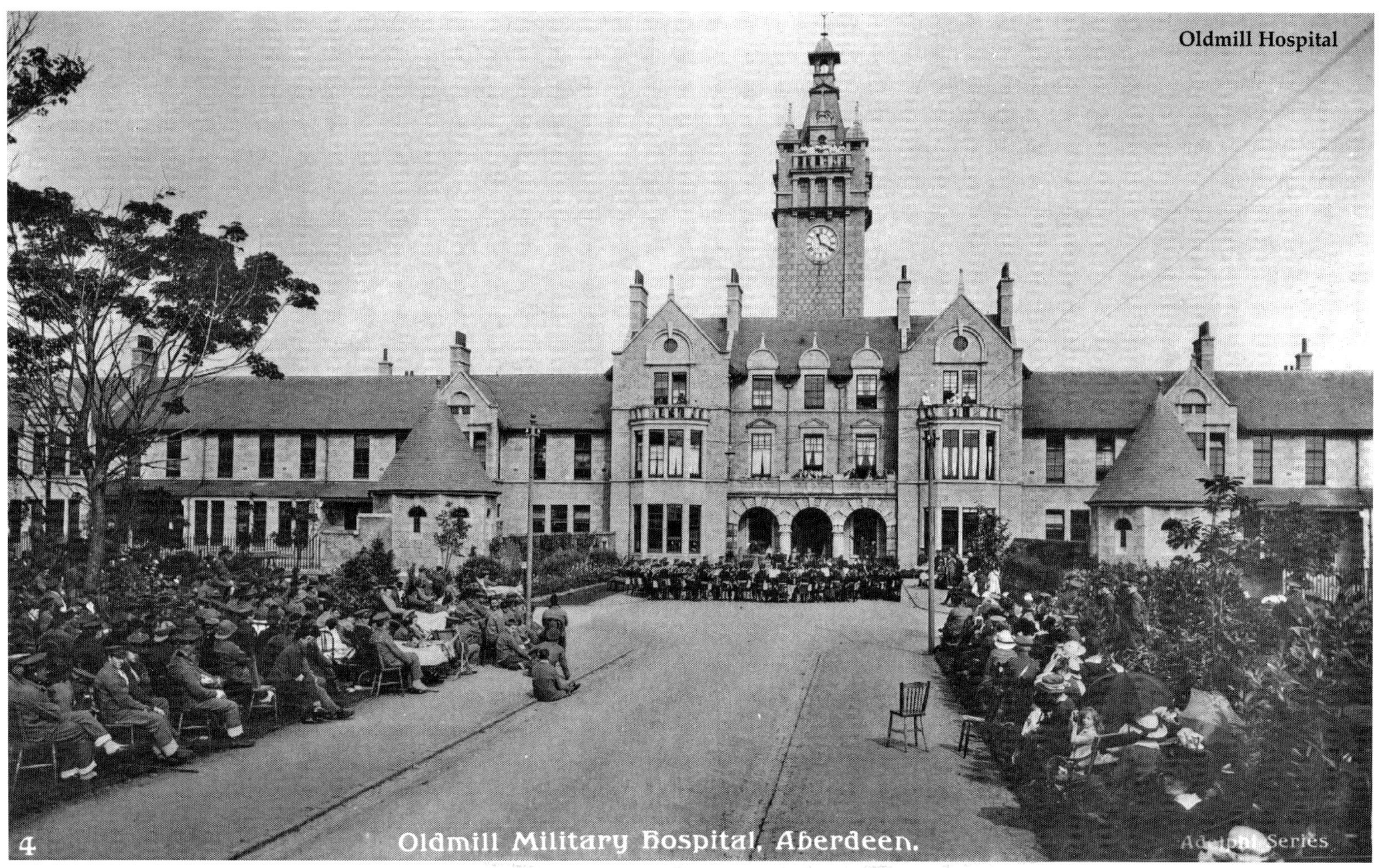


Opened by Aberdeen Parish Council as a poorhouse in 1907, one of the last to be built in Scotland, it was used as a military hospital during the First World War, when it was known as the 1st Scottish General Hospital; the postcard shows a concert in progress in front of the main entrance. The site was taken over by the town council in 1927 and became Woodend Municipal Hospital, with 225 beds caring for chronic sick and indigent poor along with some infectious disease cases. Again used by the military during the Second World War, under the National Health Service it served as a general hospital, and now cares for orthopaedics, rehabilitation and care of the elderly. The clock building is again a water tower.

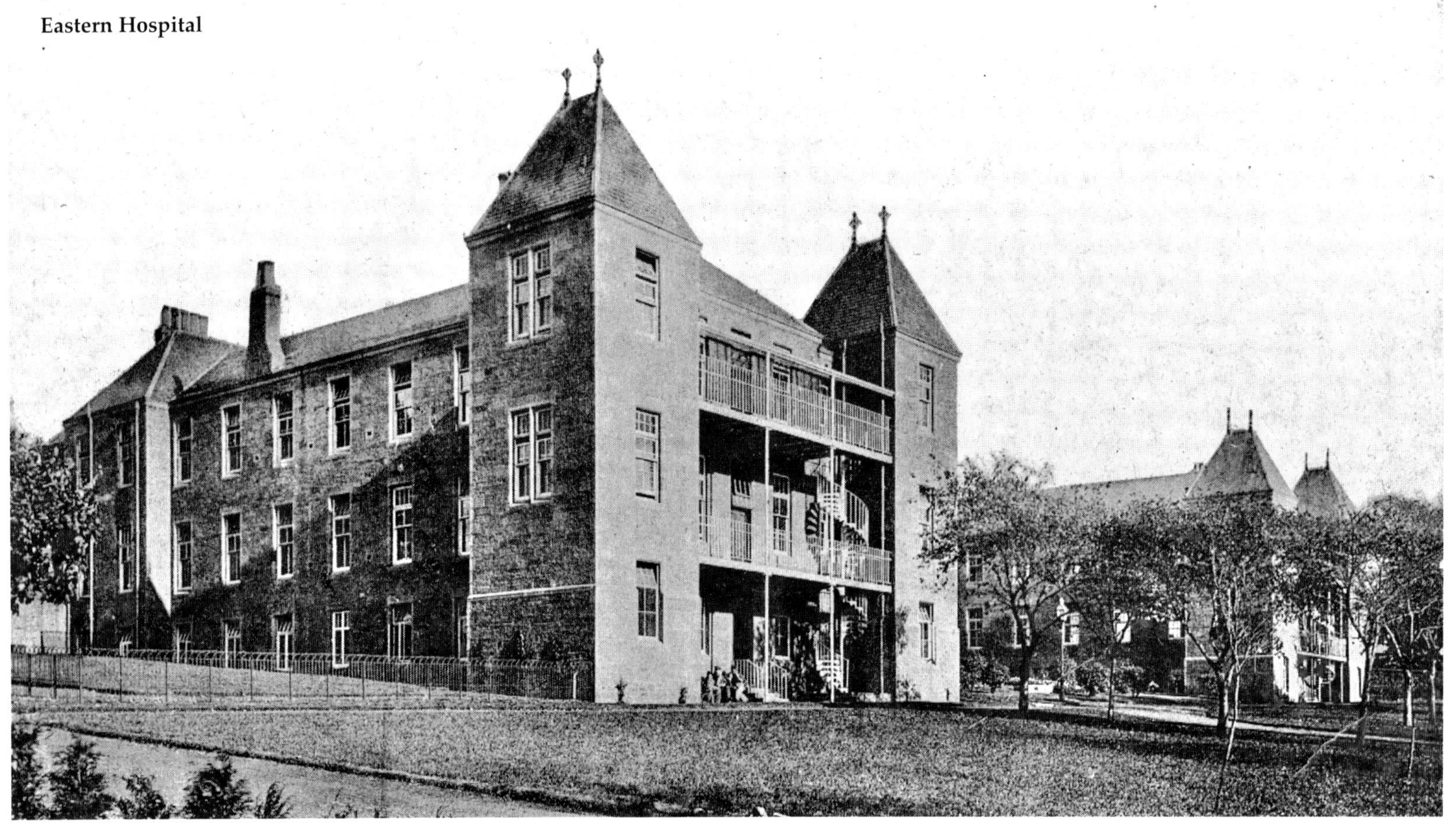

The East Poorhouse near Stobswell in Dundee opened in 1856, having been planned to house 800 paupers, 100 sick and 100 'lunatics'. Built alongside this was the Poor Law Eastern hospital, illustrated above, run by Dundee Parish Council which opened in 1893; by the Second World War this had become a municipal Maryfield hospital with accommodation for 329 patients, and 60 more were taken over from the poorhouse. Despite investments in new departments, notably maternity, child care and geriatrics after the war such that it gradually lost its Poor Law image, the building was deemed entirely unsuitable for modern Hospital purposes and patients were moved to the new Ninewells Hospital and Medical School when it opened in 1974. Maryfield Hospital was mostly demolished by 1990. The poorhouse was renamed 'the Rowans' after the inception of the NHS, but in 1977 was deemed "surplus to requirements" by the social work department. In the 1960s, a world record was set at Maryfield when a patient went 382 days without solid food, surviving on tea, coffee, soda water and vitamins, his weight falling from 214 to 80 kilograms.

# Hospitals for special purposes

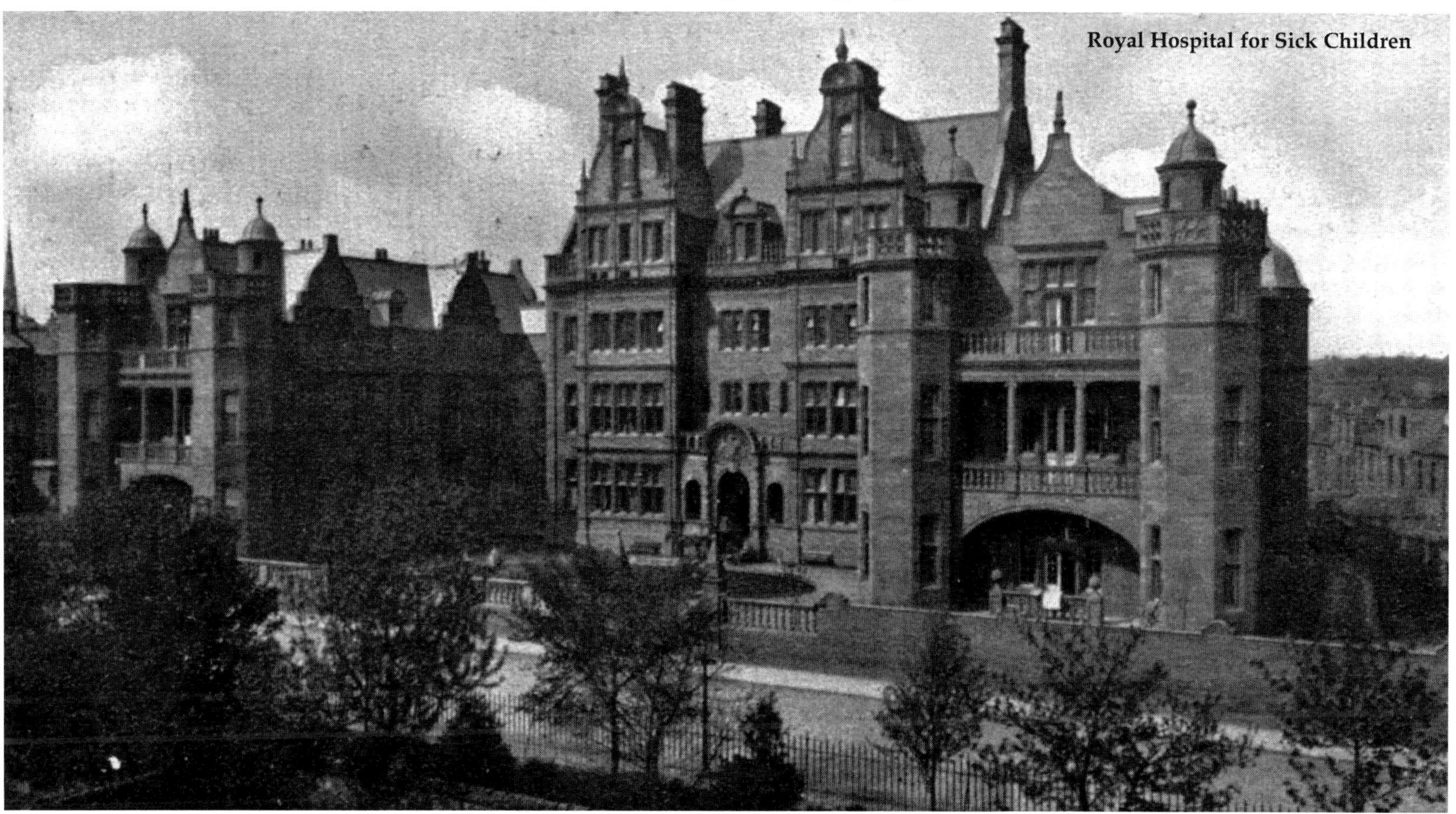

Royal Hospital for Sick Children

Opening in Lauriston Lane, Edinburgh, in 1860, the 20 bed Sick Children's Hospital gained Royal Patronage three years later, and after two changes of home moved to the George Washington Browne-designed Jacobean building on Sciennes Road in 1895. Built of red sandstone, this well-endowed and imposing hospital with 136 beds and cots was built on the site of the Trades Maiden Hospital, which was a 1704 boarding school for craftsmen's children. Caring for children from birth to around 13 years of age, the hospital continued to expand and lead the way in many aspects of paediatric medicine, and there were 210 beds by 1973. Various additions over the years made the hospital a patchwork of add-on buildings, and in order to continue providing high quality care the hospital is scheduled to move to the Royal Infirmary site with 233 beds in 2018, to be renamed the Royal Hospital for Children and Young People. The 1895 building seen here has been bought by a development firm.

## The Royal Samaritan Hospital for Women, Glasgow

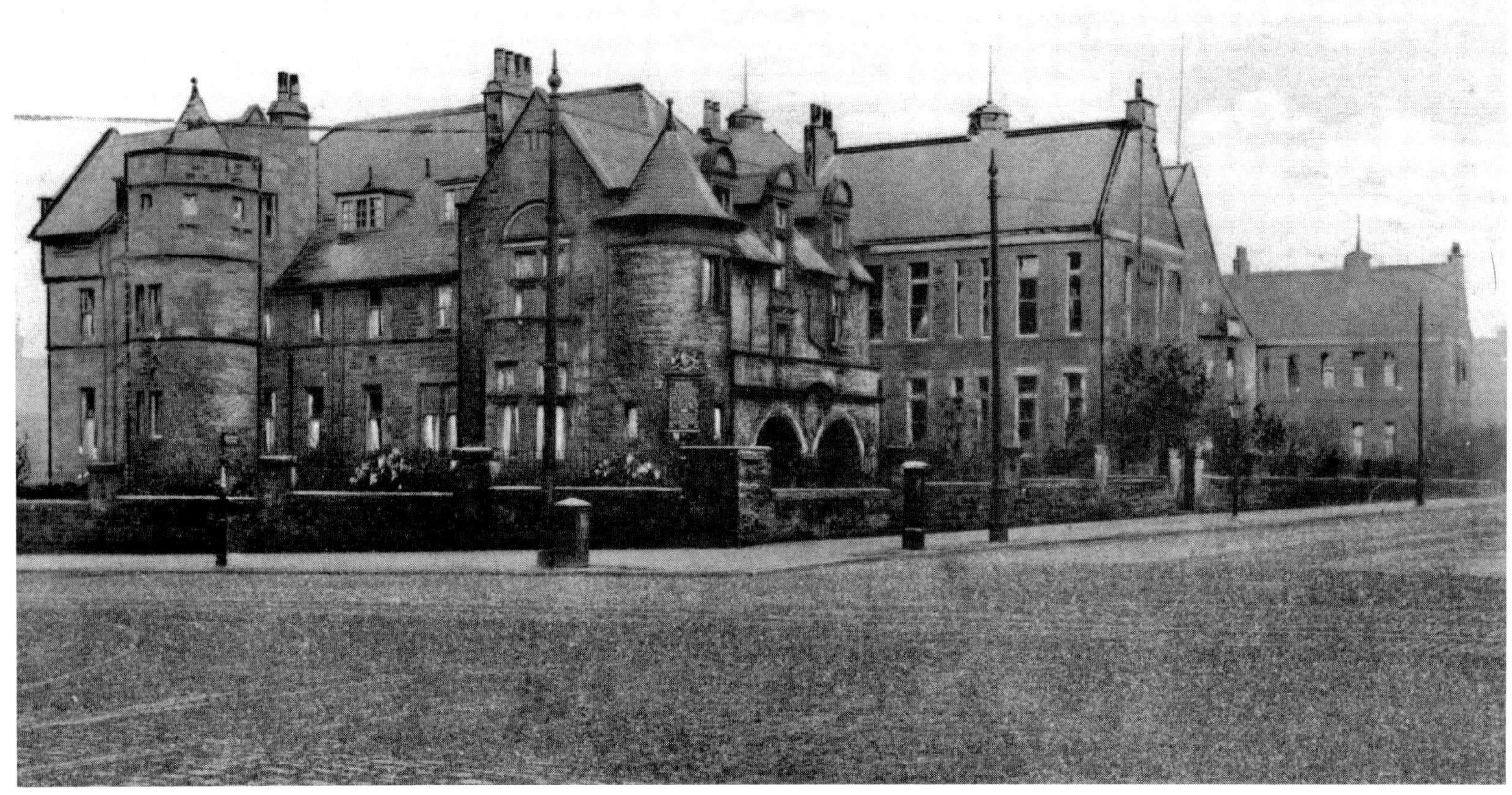

By the 1880s gynaecology as a surgical speciality was becoming more widely recognised and this hospital opened in 1886 with three beds, moving to a ten bed establishment four years later. The hospital then moved to Coplaw Street in Govanhill (as seen here) in 1896, a new purpose-built building constructed of red sandstone in a mixed style with Scottish Baronial and Art Nouveau elements, designed by MacWhannel and Rogerson; its conscious domestic character was very unusual and an early example of deliberate use of psychology in hospital design. A Royal Charter was granted in the Edwardian era, and the initial bed complement of 30 became 186 following a number of extensions by 1936. After closing in 1991, it briefly reopened the following year for orthopaedic and general surgery, and has since converted to housing and Samaritans House community hub.

# Convalescent hospitals

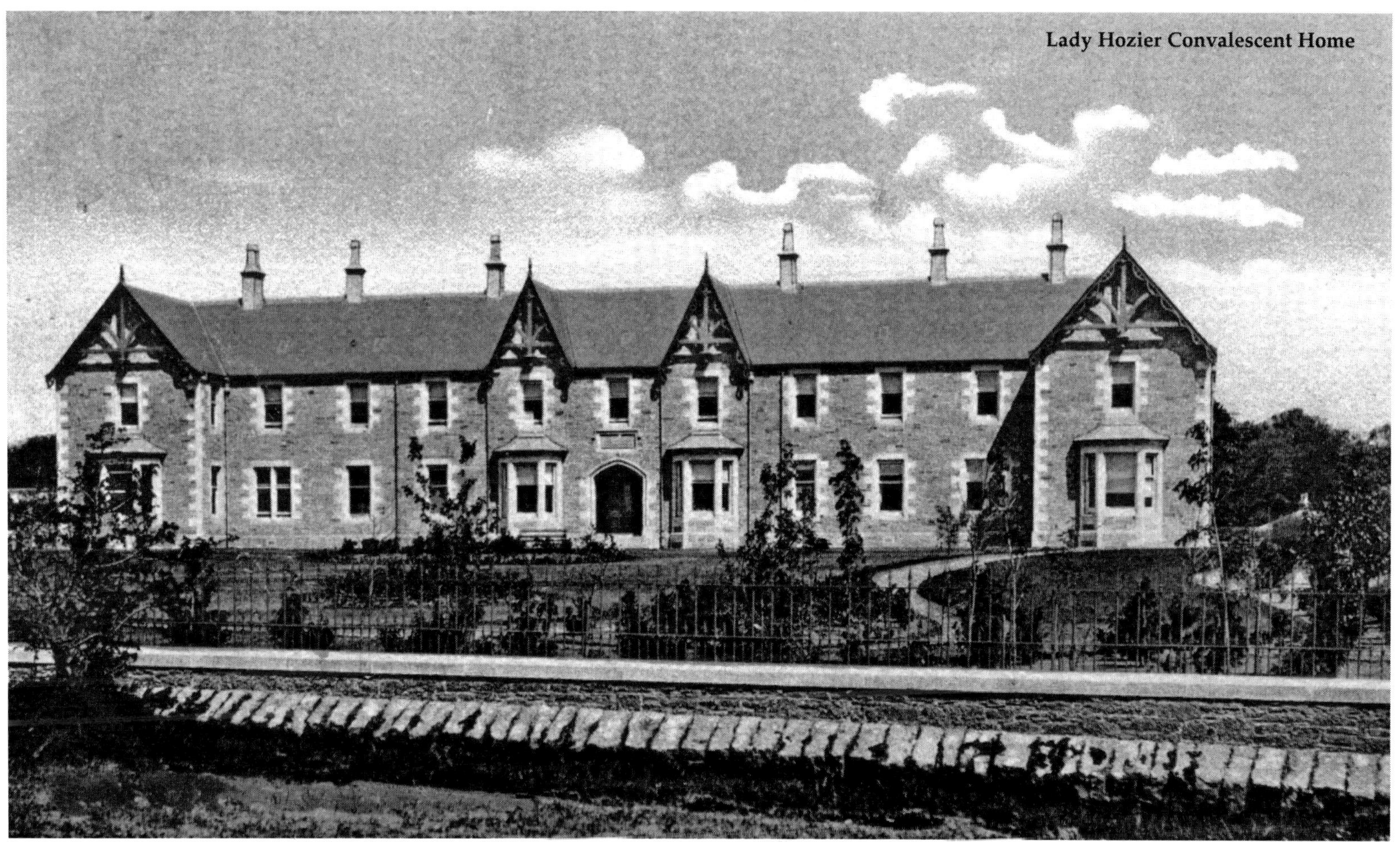

Lady Hozier Convalescent Home

Funded by Sir William Hozier of Mauldslie Castle in memory of his wife and built on the site of a redundant military barracks, Lady Hozier Convalescent Home, Lanark, opened in 1893. Conversion of the barracks proved too difficult, and a purpose-built home was eventually undertaken. The Home served Glasgow Western Infirmary and had a maximum capacity of 30 patients. It was not perhaps the choicest location, with a poorhouse and fever hospital on one side and auction mart and slaughterhouse on the other, but was operational until the early 1980s when it became a business centre.

## Convalescent Hospital, Cults

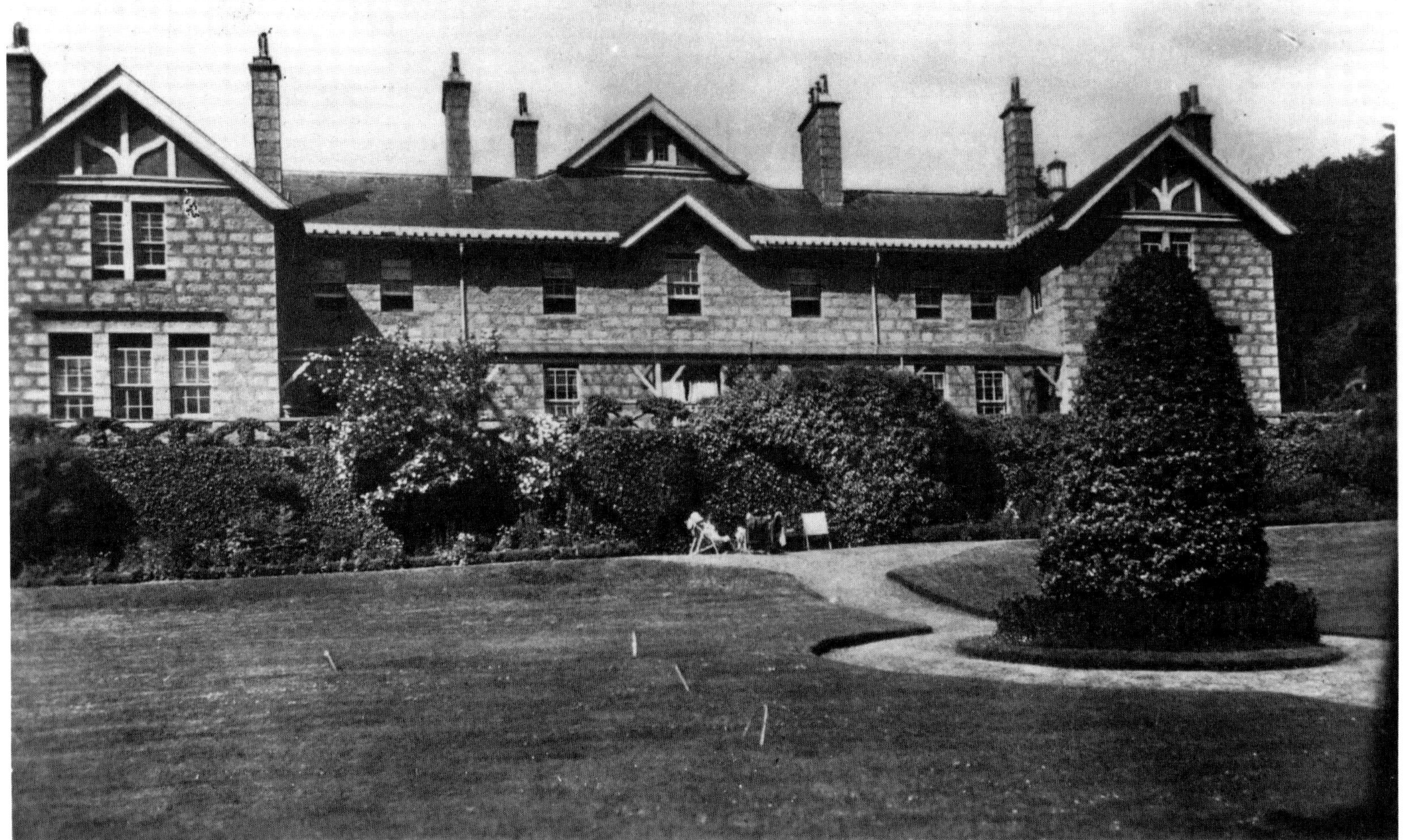

A convalescent hospital was established for Aberdeen Royal Infirmary in 1874, but although of benefit, it was largely unused and continually in debt despite receiving rental income. It was later bought by the asylum, and a decision was made to build a new convalescent hospital in Cults away from the filth of Aberdeen, this opening in 1897. Closure came in 1964 after Glen o' Dee Sanatorium became a convalescent hospital. Cults Hospital later became the Aberdeen Waldorf School.

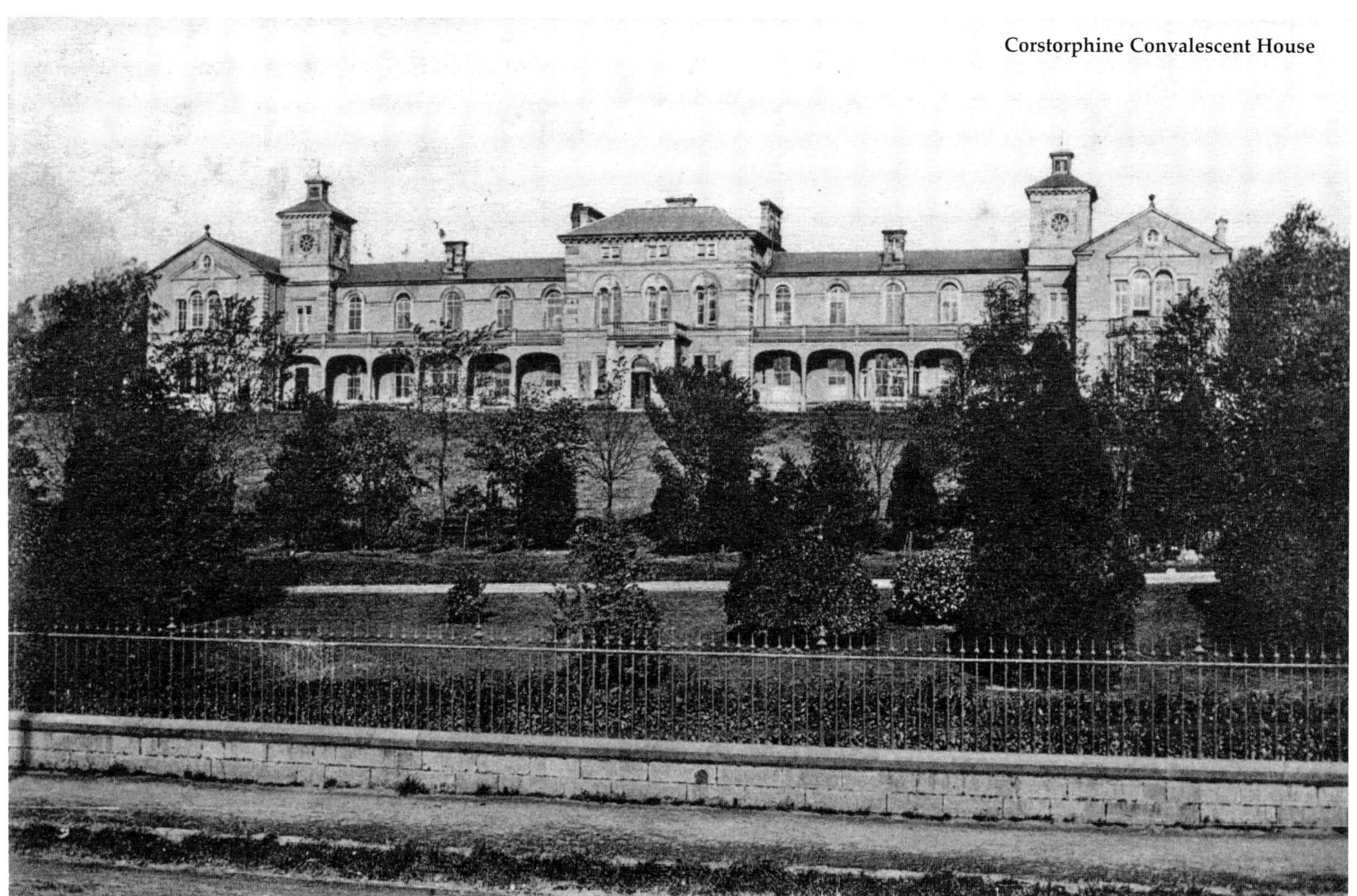

This Italianate Corstorphine Convalescent Home for Edinburgh Royal Infirmary, built to designs by Peddie and Kinnear opened in 1867 with 50 beds, with wings added on each side in 1893 increasing the bed complement to 90. In the 1960s the verandas to the front were enclosed by glass curtain walls. The convalescent house closed in 2014 and it is now a 97 bed private care home providing residential, nursing and dementia care.

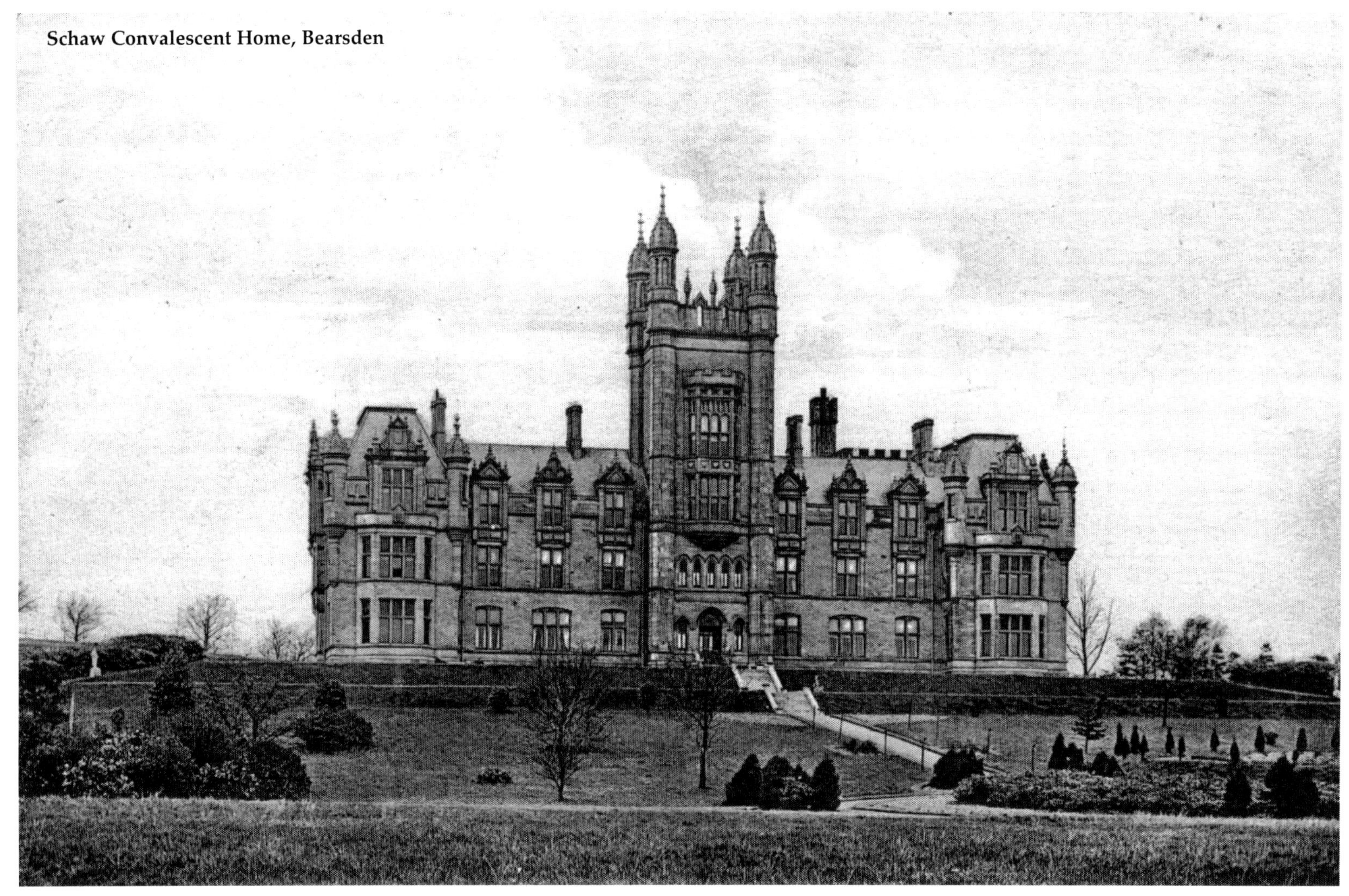

Schaw Convalescent Home, Bearsden

Built and endowed by Miss Marjorie Schaw, this convalescent home for Glasgow Royal Infirmary opened in 1895. There were 72 beds in a striking four-storey 'Tudor-Gothic' stone building with a dominating central tower. During the Second World War it was used as an 'overflow' unit for patients requiring medical attention rather than simple recuperation. After the war it was used as a geriatric hospital, and converted to private housing in 1986.

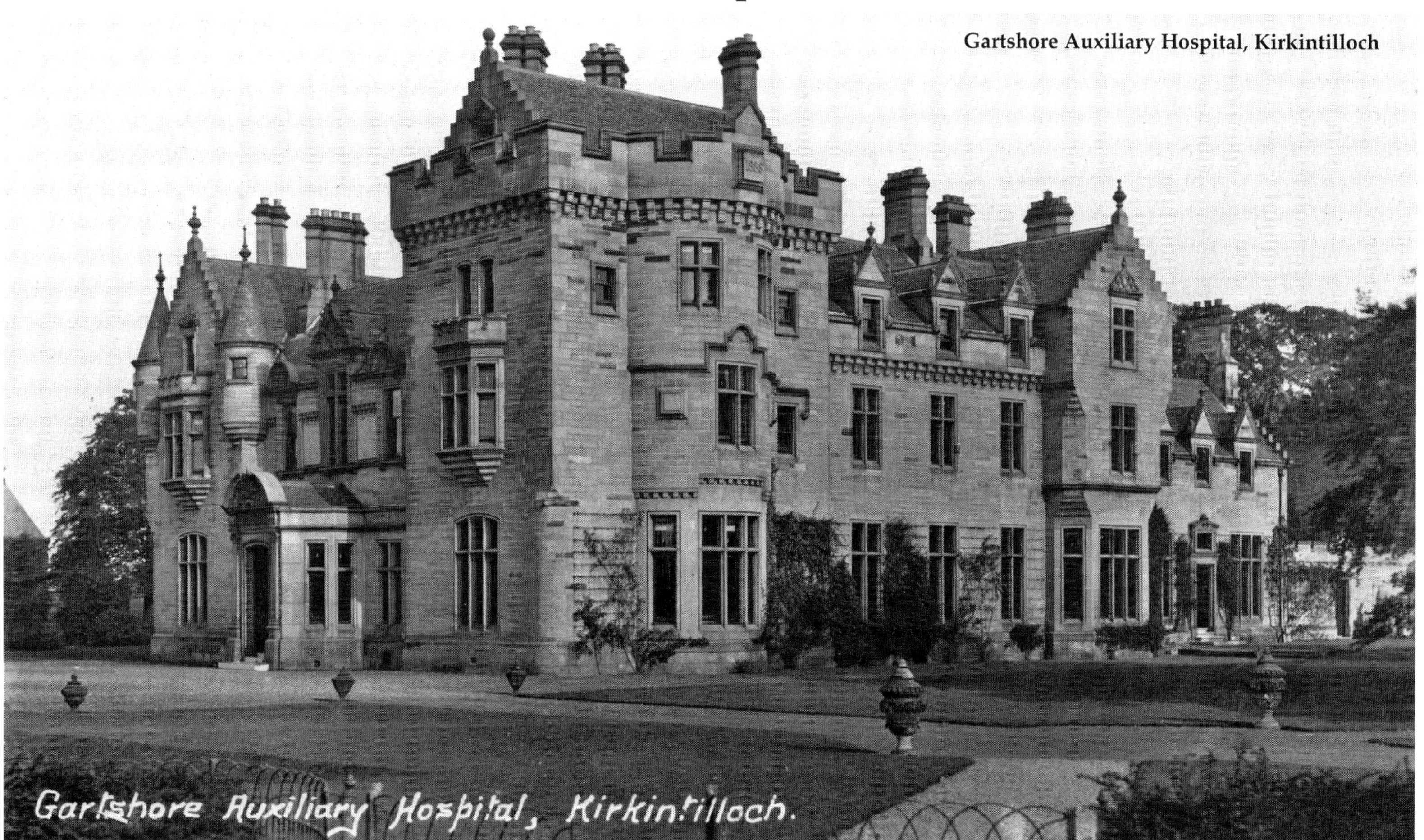


Gartshore Auxiliary Hospital, Kirkintilloch

Gartshore House was put at the disposal of the National Red Cross Society as an auxiliary hospital for wounded soldiers in the First World War, with accommodation for 150 beds. The hospital was under the management of the local Voluntary Aid Detachment (VAD) who were trained in first aid and home nursing, and began receiving patients in 1915. The government allowed 2/- per head per day for the maintenance of wounded soldiers and this was estimated to prove sufficient funds to meet the expenditure of the hospital if all the beds were occupied. In later years it was home to Viscount William Whitelaw who served in Margaret Thatcher's government.

Red Cross Hospital, Broughty Ferry
RED CROSS AUXILIARY HOSPITAL, THE LODGE, BROUGHTY FERRY

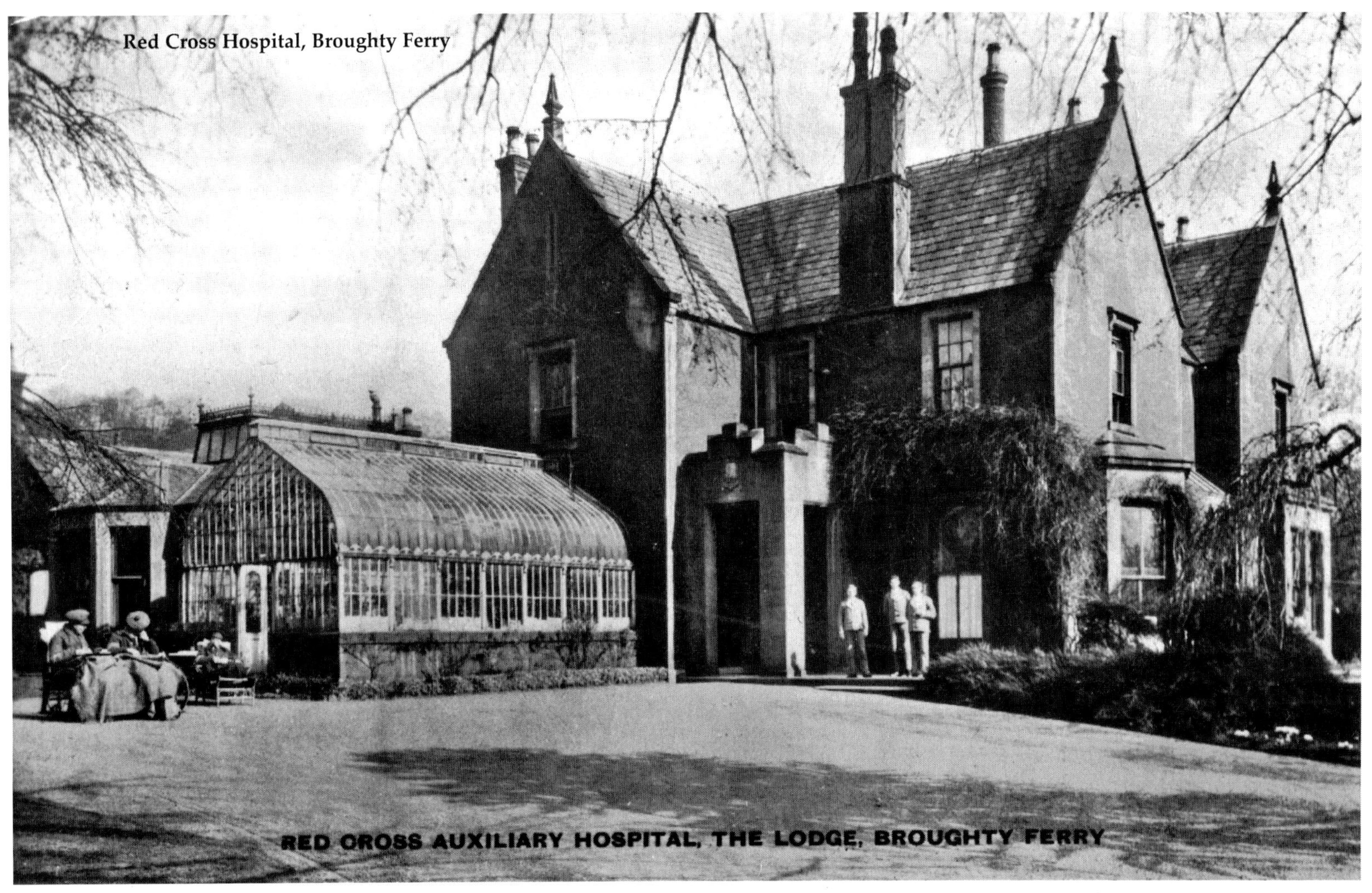

This mid 19th century house was given by the Don family in memory of the father and two sons who died during the First World War, to be used as a Red Cross Auxiliary Hospital, following which it was converted into a 40 cot infant hospital for nutritional cases. Further conversion came in 1965 when Douglas Bader, the Second World War flying ace who lost both his legs in an aerobatic accident, opened the 17 bed Dundee Limb-Fitting Centre, the first in-patient unit in the UK to offer an integrated service for amputees. This facility later moved to Ninewells Hospital and the site is now residential.

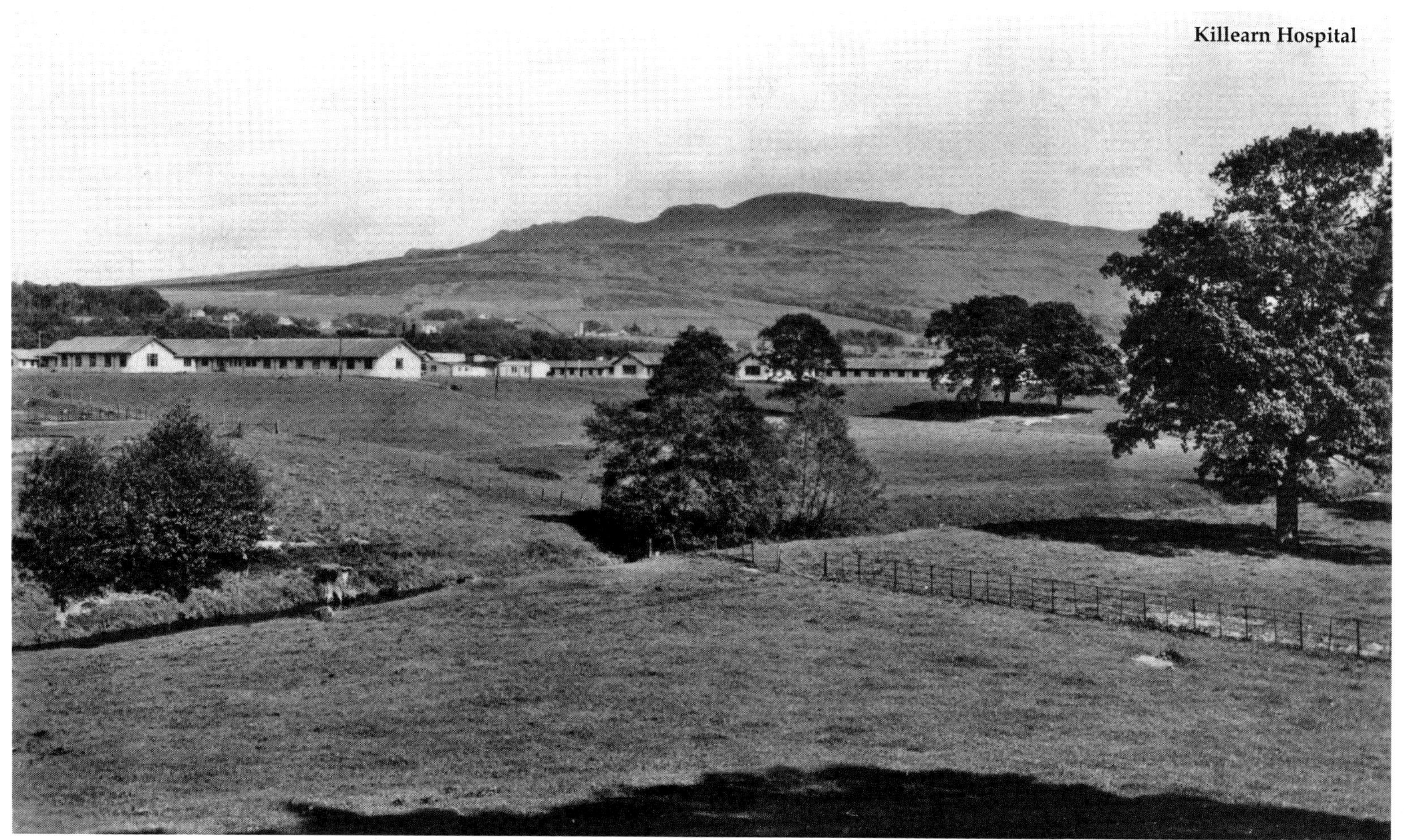

Killearn Hospital

Killearn Hospital opened in 1940 as an Emergency Medical Service hospital with 640 beds. The hospital staff were only 15 miles from Glasgow and both saw and heard the 1941 Clydebank Blitz as well as receiving casualties from it. In addition to air-raid casualties, the hospital was used for sick and wounded servicemen, injured seamen from convoys arriving in the Clyde, essential war workers and prisoners of war, as well as emergency cases from the surrounding population. After the war the bed complement reduced to 404 and the hospital became renowned for orthopaedics, peripheral nerve injury and neurosurgery specialist units. The hospital was, however, rather isolated and inconvenient, passenger rail services having been withdrawn in the 1930s, and was gradually run down, closing in 1972.

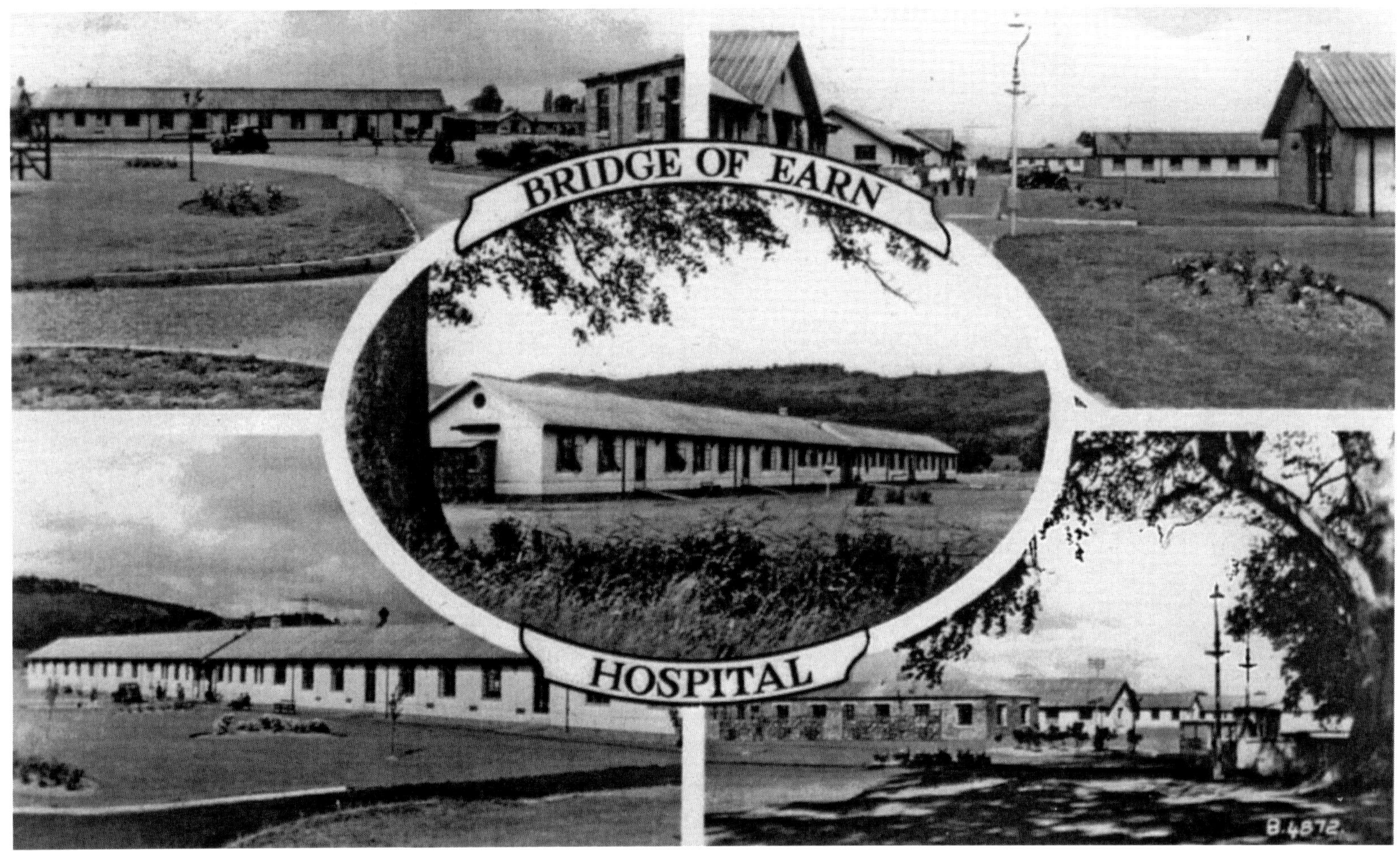


This was one of the large Emergency Medical Service hutted hospitals, built in 1940 with 1,020 beds. Expected civilian casualties did not materialise however, and initially patients came from nearby military camps, general hospitals, tuberculosis patients and prisoners of war. The busiest time for the hospital came in 1944, initially from casualties of the V1 and V2 bombing in London, and then the Normandy Invasion; by 1945, there were 1280 patients, with convoys arriving every weekend. The rehabilitation unit from Gleneagles Hotel moved here in 1946 and the orthopaedic unit from Larbert relocated the following year; these allowed Bridge of Earn to continue working after the war, and in 1973 there were 733 general beds. In 1990 there was still present much of the character of the original appearance, but the hospital closed in 1992 and was cleared in 2006 for housing.

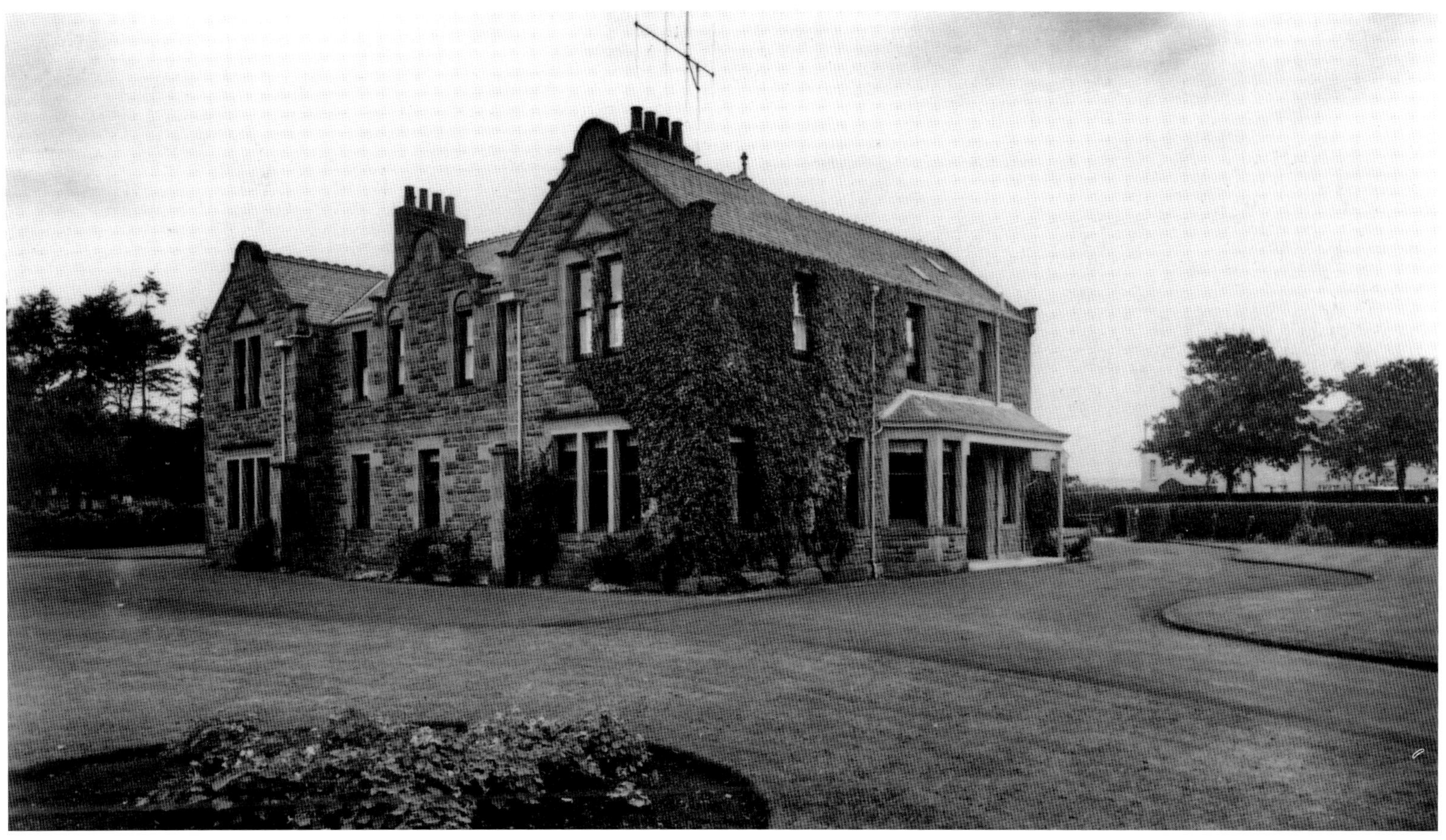

Built in Edwardian times Edzell Convalescent Home was gifted by the Johnston family of Montrose for the benefit of Montrose Royal Infirmary. The home was a handsome red sandstone building, accommodating 20 patients. During the war it was damaged by enemy action. In 1965 it became Angus House, a centre of educational excursions for local children, and in 2009 planning permission was granted for change of use to create a private dwelling.

*Back cover*: Insch and District War Memorial Hospital, Aberdeenshire, a small cottage hospital, opened with eleven beds and an operating theatre in 1922, built from public subscription as a memorial to soldiers killed in the First World War. The one storey rather cramped building took medical, major and minor surgical and maternity cases in 14 beds and four cots by wartime. The hospital benefited strongly from gifts and legacies and after the war more additions and alterations were proposed, but these fell through with the establishment of the National Health Service. There were 14 GP and maternity beds in 1973, and it is now a 15 bed community hospital.

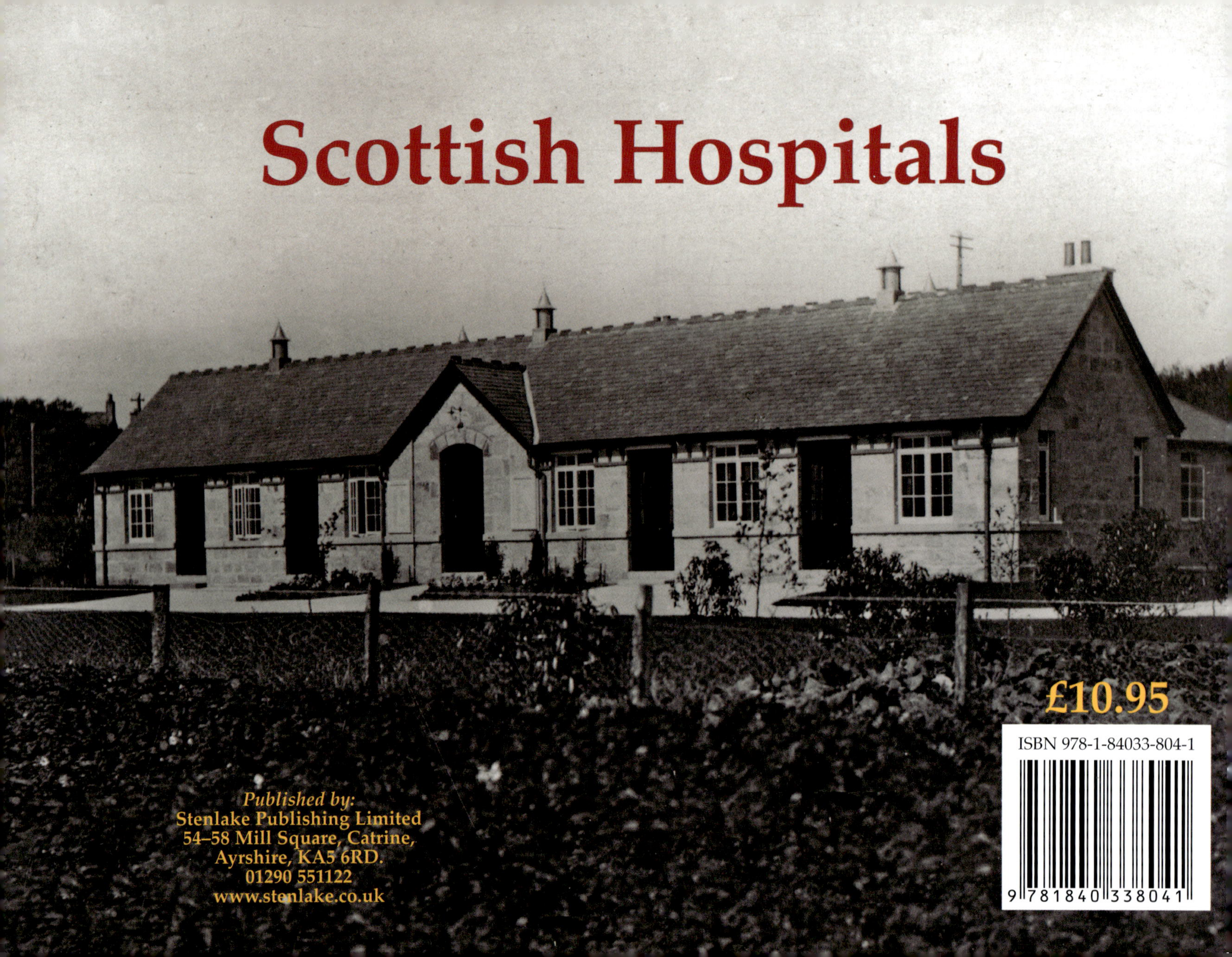

# Scottish Hospitals

£10.95

ISBN 978-1-84033-804-1

9 781840 338041

*Published by:*
**Stenlake Publishing Limited**
**54–58 Mill Square, Catrine,**
**Ayrshire, KA5 6RD.**
**01290 551122**
**www.stenlake.co.uk**